HEMOPHILIA

Edited by **Angelika Batorova**

Hemophilia
Edited by Angelika Batorova

Published by InTech
Janeza Trdine 9, 51000 Rijeka, Croatia

Publishing Process Manager Maria Radja

Technical Editor Teodora Smiljanic

Cover Designer InTech Design Team

Additional hard copies can be obtained from orders@intechopen.com

Hemophilia, Edited by Angelika Batorova
p. cm.
ISBN 978-953-51-0429-2

For EU product safety concerns:
IN TECH d.o.o., Prolaz Marije Krucifikse Kozulić 3, 51000 Rijeka, Croatia,
info@intechopen.com or visit our website at intechopen.com.

Meet the editor

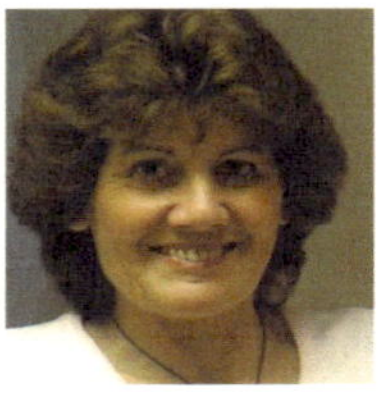

Angelika Batorova is a Medical Director of the National Hemophilia Centre and Hemostasis and Thrombosis Unit of the Department of Hematology and Transfusion Medicine, University Hospital, Bratislava.Dr Batorova received her medical education from Comenius University, Bratislava, where she specialised in the Internal Medicine,Hematology and Transfusion Medicine. In 1992 she obtained the PhD and in 2004 the position of an Associate Professor at the Medical School of the Comenius University and at the Postgraduate Medical School, both in Bratislava. The fellowship and visiting appointments included the National Hemophilia Centre in Tel Aviv , the New York Blood Center, and the Hemophilia Comprehensive Care Centers in New York. Dr Batorova´s fields of interests is the optimization of hemophilia treatment, including the treatment of inhibitors, management of surgery, continuous infusion of coagulation factors as well as the comprehensive care for congenital factor VII deficiency. Dr Batorova has worked as a member of the Executive Committee and the Medical Advisory Board of the World Federation of Hemophilia 2006-2010 and currently she is a member of the Data and Demographic Committee of the WFH and the Medical Advisory Group of the European Haemophilia Consortium.

Contents

Preface

Hemophilia is one of the longest known diseases in the history of medicine with a first description as a hereditary bleeding disorder in Talmud as early as the second century AD. However, it took many centuries until the start of modern history of disease which dates from the beginning of the 20th century. Expansion of the knowledge on the pathophysiology of the blood coagulation led to discovery of the lack of factor VIII or factor IX as a cause of the disease. The development of the blood transfusion medicine was the main prerequisite for the introduction of effective treatment of bleeding, which resides in the replacement of the missing coagulation factors. In the course of the last century, severe hemophilia has changed from potentially fatal disease having a life expectancy of only 11 years to a well treatable bleeding disorder with a life expectancy now almost approaching the value of the general population.

Significant progress towards optimum management of the disease has been achieved over the last decades, including the specialized multidisciplinary comprehensive care, home therapy and prophylaxis, employment of safe viraly inactivated plasma derived factor concentrates and most recently expanding use of recombinant factor VIII/IX concentrates. The quality of life of persons with hemophilia has dramatically improved, enabling their full implementation in professional and social life.

Major advances have been achieved in the field of molecular biology of hemophilia, which were succesfully implemented into a clinical practice, including genetic counselling, detection of hemophilia carriers, prenatal diagnosis as well as the study of genotype -phenotype relationships. Despite promising advances in genetic bioengineering the definite cure of the hemophilia is not yet available and an effective treatment requires frequent injections of factor VIII/IX concentrates. Due to this fact the research has currently focused on the development of factor VIII/IX products with prolonged biological efficacy.

There are still many challenging issues in the field of hemophilia, some of them have been discussed in the articles presented in this book. Comprehensive molecular diagnosis of hemophilia is demanding and still not widely available in many countries. However, the articles in this book demonstrate the advances in this field achieved in the research laboratories from different regions of the world. The issue of viral infections from previous era of hemophilia therapy is still actual in older

generation of hemophiliacs. The value of HCV genotyping in peripheral blood mononuclear cells for the prediction of the response to antiviral therapy in HCV infected patients with hemophilia has been discussed. In the present era of availability of safe products for the treatment of hemophilia, the development of inhibitory antibodies against factors FVIII and IX is the most challenging complication of hemophilia, requiring an alternative hemostatic therapy. This issue has been discussed in the articles on inhibitors, including the presentation of novel bypassing agent under the development. Another important issue is increasing age of hemophilia population, which has brought new requirements for the management of the health problems typical for the older adult age, especially cardiovascular, systemic and malignant diseases. The main aspects of hemophilia ageing as well as a need and/or feasibility of prophylaxis in adults has also been discussed.

This book demonstrates the great efforts aimed at further improving the care of the hemophilia, which may bring further improvement in the quality of life of hemophilia persons and their families.

I would like to thank all contributors, and especially to Marija Radija for her outstanding assistance in the compillation of this book.

Angelika Batorova
Medical Director of the National Hemophilia Centre and Hemostasis and Thrombosis
Unit of the Department of Hematology and Transfusion Medicine
University Hospital, Bratislava
Slovakia

1

Profiling of Mutations in the *F8* and *F9*, Causative Genes of Hemophilia A and Hemophilia B

Sung Ho Hwang[1], Hee-Jin Kim[2] and Hye Sun Kim[1]
[1]*Department of Biological Science, College of Natural Sciences, Ajou University, Suwon*
[2]*Department of Laboratory Medicine & Genetics, Samsung Medical Center*
Sungkyunkwan University, School of Medicine, Seoul
Republic of Korea

1. Introduction

Hemophilia, a common congenital coagulation disorder, is classified as hemophilia A (HA) and hemophilia B (HB), which result from a deficiency or dysfunction of coagulation factor VIII (FVIII) and factor IX (FIX), respectively. HA is known to be caused by heterogeneous mutations of the FVIII gene (*F8*), such as inversions, substitutions, deletions, insertions, etc. *F8* (NM_000132.3) is located on the long arm of the Xq28 region of the X chromosome. *F8* is extremely large (186 kb) and consists of 26 exons (Graw et al., 2005). The transcript of *F8* is approximately 9010 bp and comprises a short 5′-untranslated region (5′-UTR; 150 bp), an open reading frame (ORF) plus stop codon (7056 bp), and a long 3′-UTR (1806 bp). The protein product of *F8* is a cofactor of FIX, without enzyme activity. The ORF encodes a signal peptide with 19 amino acids at its N-terminus, which leads to the passage of FVIII through hepatocytes to blood vessels. The matured FVIII protein contains 2332 amino acids and a glycoprotein of approximately 250 kDa, and circulates as an inactive pro-cofactor.

FVIII is a multi-domain protein composed of A1-A2-B-A3-C1-C2, named from the N-terminus. FVIII synthesized in hepatocytes is secreted into the circulation and readily assembled with von Willebrand factor (vWF), which is generated and secreted by endothelial cells. Besides vWF, FVIII protein can also interact with diverse proteins such as thrombin and FX. These interactions are important for effective hemostasis. However, *F8* mutations can lead to the production of truncated proteins, which lead to disruption of FVIII function and suppress normal protein interaction with proteins involved in the coagulation cascade (Bowen, 2002). This inappropriate reaction causes bleeding tendency.

F8 mutations can occur at diverse sites in a variety of types, such as structural variation (inversions of intron 22 or intron 1) and sequence variation (insertion, deletion, and substitution). The latter variation leads to nonsense, missense, and frameshift mutations. Recently, more than 1,200 types of *F8* mutations were reported in the HAMSTeRS (Hemophilia A Mutation, Structure, Test and Resource Site) database (http://hadb.org.uk).

The *F9* gene (NM_000133.3) is also located on the X chromosome at Xq27.1–q27.2. In contrst to *F8*, the size of *F9* gene is approximately 34 kb with only eight exons and the size of the transcript mRNA is 2803 bp. The *F9* gene encodes the FIX protein, one of the vitamin

K-dependent coagulation factors in humans. FIX is synthesized in the liver as 461 amino acid residues, including 46 signal peptides at its N-terminus. It circulates in the blood as a single-chain glycoprotein of inactive zymogen (Yoshitake et al., 1985). When coagulation is initiated, FIX is converted to an active form (FIXa) by proteolytic cleavage, resulting in an N-terminal light chain and a C-terminal heavy chain held together by one or more disulfide bonds (Di Scipio et al., 1978; Lindquist et al., 1978). The role of FIXa in the blood coagulation cascade is to activate factor X through interactions with calcium ions, membrane phospholipids, and FVIII.

More than 1,000 mutations have been reported for *F9* to date (http://hadb.org.uk). The data archived in the locus-specific mutation database for *F9* (http://www.kcl.ac.uk/ip/petergreen/haemBdatabase.html) describe the genotype-phenotype correlations. Although the mutations are scattered over the entire structure of the *F9* gene, the distribution of mutation types shows that missense/nonsense mutations are the most common, accounting for ~64% of mutations, followed by frameshift mutations (~17%). More than 90% of mutations are point mutations that can be detected by direct sequencing analyses (Mahajan et al., 2007). The rest (<10%) consist of large exon deletion mutations or complex rearrangements. Unlike in HA, mutations with large inversion rearrangement are rare in HB.

2. Profiling of the *F8* mutations

The profiling of *F8* mutations is important for a precise diagnosis of HA, understanding of genotype-phenotype correlation, carrier detection, prenatal diagnosis, and predicting inhibitor development. As there are various types of mutations, we propose a strategy for profiling *F8* mutations as follows (Figure 1)

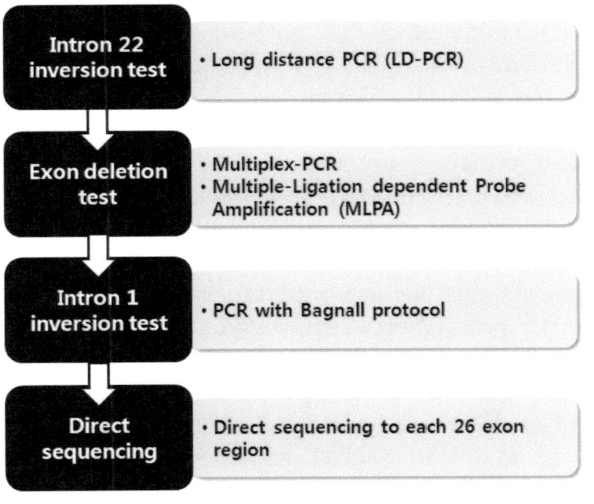

Fig. 1. A proposed strategy for profiling of *F8* mutation.

2.1 Identification of inversions in intron 22 or intron 1

The most common defect in *F8* is intron 22 inversion, which occurs via homologous recombination between *int22h-1* (intragenic) with *int22h-2* or *int22h-3* (extragenic) (Liu et al.,

1998). Figure 2 is a schematic presentation of intron 22 inversion of *F8*. The incidence of intron 22 inversion is approximately 40~50% in severe HA patients, and without a significant ethnic difference (Bowen, 2002). Intron 22 inversion is also a high risk factor for inhibitor formation, thus, it has drawn special attention as a hotspot of *F8* mutation (Oldenburg et al., 2000; Oldenburg et al., 2002). In a previous report, HA patients with intron 22 inversion exhibited an inhibitor prevalence of >22% (Boekhorst et al., 2008). For this reason, tests for intron 22 inversion have been the primary step of *F8* mutation profiling.

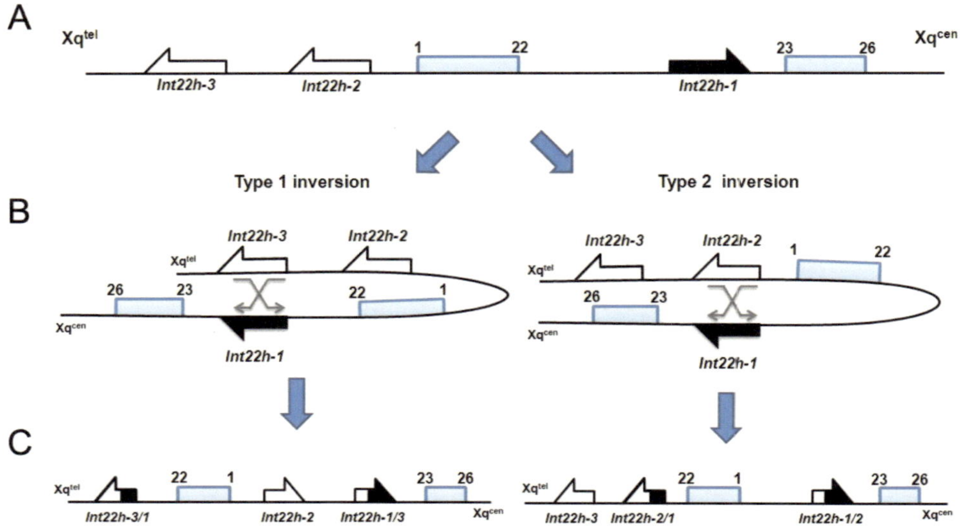

Fig. 2. Schematic presentation of the intron 22 inversion of the *F8*. (A) The normal structure of the *F8* gene. Gray boxes represent exon region and upper number is exon number. White arrow represent intron 22 homologous region (*int22h-2*; proximal and *int22h-3*; distal region) and black arrow indicates *int22h-1* (intragenic). (B) Homologous recombination process occurs between *int22h-1* and *int22h-2* (type 2 inversion) or *int22h-3* (type 1 inversion). (C) The inversions induce disruption of *F8* gene. Exons 1 to 22 are displaced towards the telomere and are oriented in a direction opposite to their normal orientation.
Xq^{tel}: X- chromosome q arm telomere, Xq^{cen}: X-chromosome q arm centromere.

Recently, the long-distance PCR (LD-PCR) method was developed for more effective investigation of intron 22 inversion (Liu et al., 1998; Polakova et al., 2003). LD-PCR is conducted with primers P, Q, A, and B in accordance with the methods of Liu *et al* (1998). Primers are designed so that primers P and Q bind to *int22h-1*, whereas primers A and B bind to *int22h-2* and *int22h-3* (Figures 3A and 3B). Figure 3C illustrates an LD-PCR result identifying a Korean HA patient with intron 22 inversion. Lanes 1, 4, and 7 indicate the product of the A+B primer pair (10 kb), which was amplified in both the inversion positive and negative patients. However, there was a difference between the B+P primer pair product in the intron 22 inversion and the wild type; an 11 kb product was generated only in the inversion patient (lanes 5 and 8) but not in the wild type (lane 2). Additionally, the result of the product from P+Q showed that a 12 kb band was generated only in the wild type (lane 3) but not in the inversion patient (lanes 6 and 9). These results demonstrate that the LD-PCR is an effective method for the identification of intron 22 inversion HA patients.

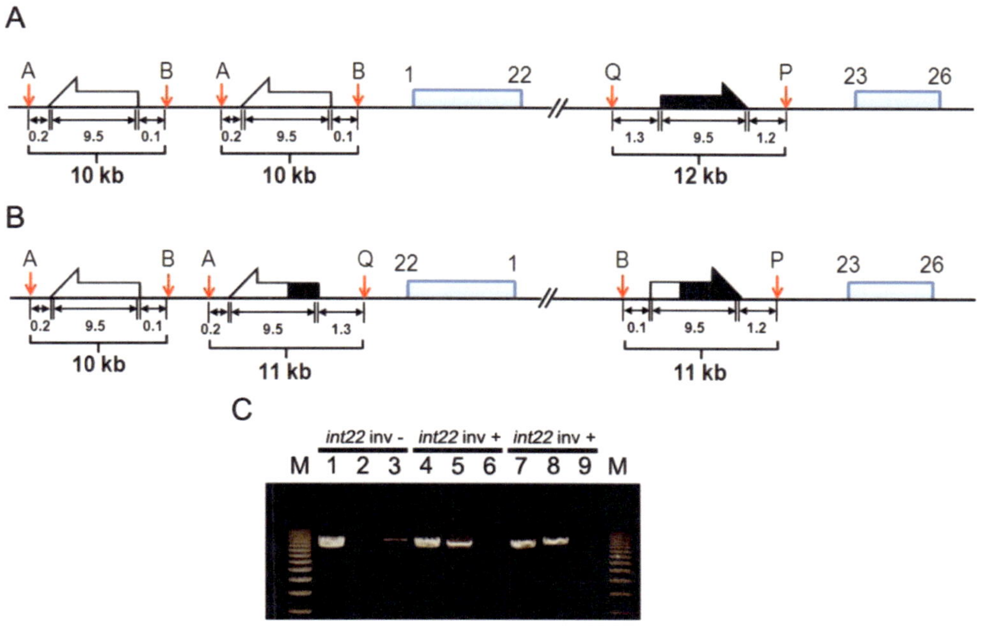

Fig. 3. Primer design for LD-PCR and result of intron 22 inversion test . (A) The normal formation of *F8* gene and intron 22 homologous region and (B) intron 22 inversion-occured *F8* gene. Red arrows represent binding sites for the primers A, B, P and Q. Primers A and B hybridize to forward and rear region of *int22h-2* and *int22h-3*. Combination of primers P and Q hybridize to forward and rear region of *int22h-1*. In the inversion-negative case, LD-PCR with the primers A+B will make a 10 kb PCR product and primers P+Q make a 12 kb one. However, primer B+P will not make any PCR product. While inversion-positive patient will produce a 11 kb band with the primer B+P mixture. (C) Intron 22 inversion test by LD-PCR to one intron 22-negative and two intron 22-positive patients. Lanes 1, 4 and 7 show the results of the primer A+B (product size is a 10 kb) which is amplified in both the inversion and non-inversion cases. Lanes 2, 5 and 8 show the product of the primer B+P mixture for the detection of inversion (11 kb). Lanes 3, 6 and 9 indicate the product of the P+Q primer mixture. M indicates size marker.

Keeney et al (2005) recently reported that multiplex-PCR is available for carrier detection. The multiplex-PCR reaction for the detection of intron 22 inversion is conducted with primers A+B+P+Q combined in 1 tube. If a sister is a HA carrier with intron 22 inversion, 3 bands (10 kb, 11 kb, and 12 kb) will be produced. However, if a sister does not have an intron 22 inversion mutation, the products will be 2 (10 kb and 12 kb) rather than 3 bands.

Similar to intron 22 inversion, intron 1 inversion also occurs via homologous recombination between *int1h-1* (intragenic) and *int1h-2* (extragenic) in the *F8* promoter region (Bagnall et al., 2002). Figure 4 represents a schematic of homologous recombination in *int1h-1* and *int1h-2*. In the figure, homologous recombination will result in an intron 1 breaking inversion and induces a severe mutation. Although several studies have investigated the prevalence of intron 1 inversion, its prevalence remains controversial (1~5% in HA) (Schroder, J. et al.,

2006). The importance of intron 1 inversion is also related to inhibitor formation (Fidanci et al., 2008; Repesse et al., 2007).

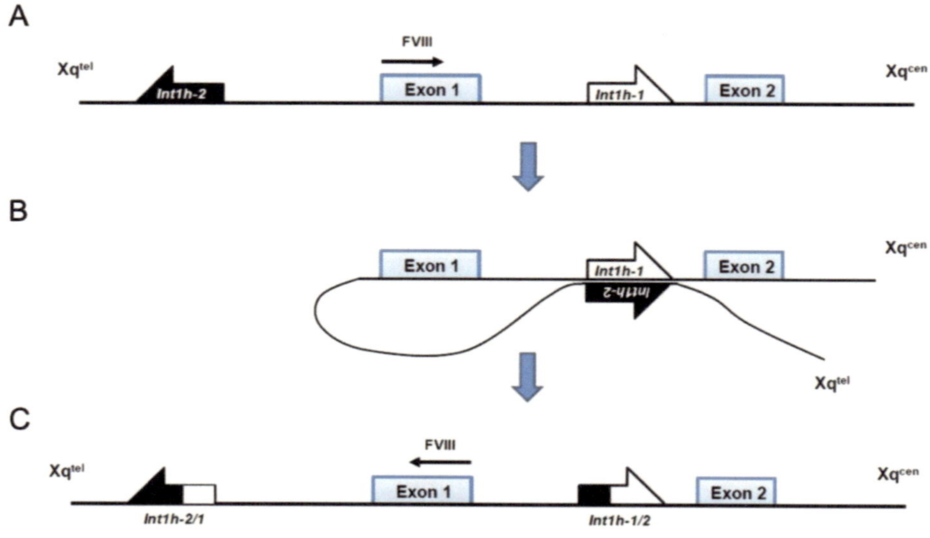

Fig. 4. Scehmatic veiw of intron 1 inversion process. (A) Homologous region of intron 1 is located in the intragenic region (white arrow, *int1h-1*) and extragenic region (black arrow, *int1h-2*). (B) Homologous recombination occurs between *int1h-1* and *int1h-2*. (C) The result of intron 1 inversion will not synthesize an appropriated FVIII protein because the direction of expression is changed. $Xq^{tel:}$ X- chromosome q arm telomere, Xq^{cen}: X-chromosome q arm centromere.

To profile *F8* mutations, we investigated intron 22 inversion and exon deletion (to be discussed later) and then the patients without intron 22 inversion and exon deletion were tested for intron 1 inversion. The amplification products of *int1h-1* and *int1h-2* are analyzed with the method described by Bagnall et al (2002). For detection of intron 1 inversion, primers 9F, 9cF, 2F, and 2R were prepared according to the guidelines established by Bagnall et al (Figure 5). The mixed primers 9cR+9F+2F and 2F+2R+9F were used for the amplification of *int1h-1* and *int1h-2*, respectively. The product of primers 9cR+9F+2F (*int22h-1*) was expected to be a 2.0 kb band, whereas the primers 2F+2R+9F (*int22h-2*) were expected to generate a 1.2 kb product from the wild-type sample (Figure 5A). As shown in Figure 5C, 1.4 kb and 1.8 kb amplicons were produced by the 2F+9F+9cR primers and 2F+2R+9F primers (lanes 1 and 2), respectively, in the case of intron 1 inversion. However, the wild type (inversion test negative) produced 2.0 kb and 1.2 kb PCR products (Figure 5C, lane 3 and lane 4).

2.2 Identification of exon deletion by multiplex-PCR method

Although direct sequencing is a useful method for detection of sequence variation, it has been reported that the method is unable to detect certain gross exon deletions (El-Maarri et al., 2005). For this reason, investigation for gross exon deletion is needed for *F8* mutation profiling before sequence analysis can be carried out. In a previous study, we reported identifying a HA patient with gross exon deletion by applying multiplex-PCR. We designed 35 primers to

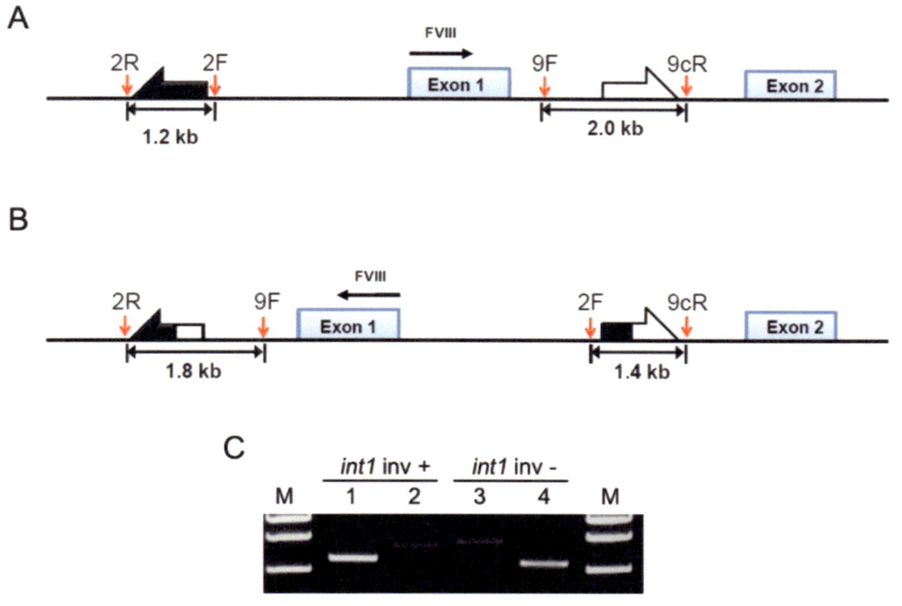

Fig. 5. Primer design and intron 1 inversion test. Linearised diagram of normal (A) and intron 1 inversion (B) of *F8* gene. Red arrows indicate binding sites for each primer. (C) The result of intron 1 inversion test. Primer 2F+9F+9cR combination (lane 1, 3) and primer 2F+2R+9F combination (lane 2, 4) were used for the amplifications of *int1h-1* and *int1h-2*, respectively. (C) Lane 1 and 2 illustrate the product of the intron 1 inversion-positive patient, whereas lane 3 and 4 illustrate intron 1 inversion- negative patients. M: 1 kb size marker.

detect the 26 exons of *F8* (Hwang et al., 2009). In contrast to the routinely used singleplex PCR, which requires 35 PCR reactions per patient to detect exon deletion, only 8 PCR reactions were necessary when multiplex-PCR was used (Figure 6). These results demonstrate that multiplex-PCR is simple and useful for many PCR product analyses in 1-tube reactions. As exon deletion tends to be associated with severe phenotypes, a detection method with simple and accurate application is very important. This method is easily applied to PCR machines and requires no special equipment such as a capillary sequencer for multiplex ligation-dependent probe amplification (MLPA) (Lannoy et al., 2009). Although the MLPA method is powerful and has its advantages, such as being free from primer dimerization and false priming, multiplex-PCR is still a useful method for the detection of exon deletion in local laboratories or in developing countries. Thus, multiplex-PCR analysis can be used as the secondary test prior to direct sequencing. We found that the incidence of gross exon deletion in the Korean HA was 2.6% (Hwang et al 2009).

2.3 Direct sequencing analysis

Finally, direct sequencing can be applied to patients who do not have the mutations mentioned above. In many reports, there is no hotspot for the distribution of sequence variations in *F8* (Bogdanova et al., 2005; Tuddenham et al., 1994). Therefore, all 26 exons, including splicing sites and some portions of the intron region, should be covered by

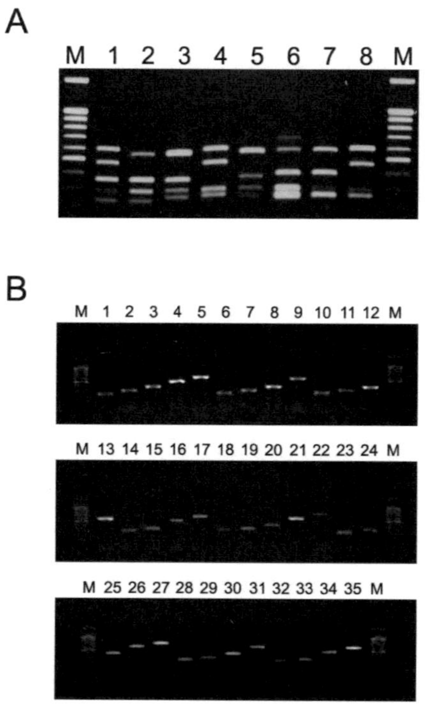

Fig. 6. Detection of gross exon deletion by multiplex-PCR. (A) Multiplex-PCR were performed with 8 primer sets. (B) Singleplex-PCR was performed with 35 primers. The numbers on each lane indicates the primer set (1~8) and single primer (lane 1~35). M: 100 bp size marker.

sequencing analysis. One of the more useful primer sequences is the set developed by David et al (David et al., 1994). These primers contain approximately 20 nucleotides of intronic sequences flanking each exon. The mRNA sequence of *F8* was used for the detection of mutations at splicing sites because certain splicing site mutations are not detected when genomic DNA material is used (Chao et al., 2003; El-Maarri et al., 2005). Conformational sensitive gel electrophoresis (CSGE) or denaturing gradient gel electrophoresis (DGGE) is applied for the detection of mutations with single or larger base mismatches (Korkko et al., 1998). The assay is based on the assumption that a buffer containing mild denaturing solvents can resolve the conformational changes produced by single-base matches in double-strand DNA, which result in an increase of the differential migration in electrophoresis (Korkko et al., 1998). However, these methods are very sensitive to experimental conditions; thus, optimization of conditions is a difficult and time-consuming process. As the cost of sequencing analysis is decreasing by the day, we applied sequencing analysis to each PCR product with reference to the *F8* sequence (NM_000132.3) and without mutation screening by CSGE or DGGE. The results of sequencing were analyzed with diverse programs such as DNASTAR, CLC workbench, and ClusteralW. We identified various sequence variations from Korean HA patients who did not have the mutations mentioned above. These mutations included 8 novel types that were not listed in the HAMSTeRS database (Hwang et al., 2009)

3. Profiling of the *F9* mutation

The identification of disease-causing mutations in the *F9* gene is also critical for diagnosis, genotype-phenotype correlations including inhibitor risk, genetic counseling, and prenatal diagnosis of HB. (Mahajan et al., 2007; Tagariello et al., 2007). More than 1,000 mutations have been reported in the literature, and the distribution of mutation types in HB is somewhat different from those in HA (HGMD Professional 2010.4, release date 18 December 2010, URL: http://www.hgmd.org/). A locus-specific mutation database also exists for HB (The Hemophilia B Mutation Database - version 13, last update in 2004, URL: http://www.kcl.ac.uk/ip/petergreen/haemBdatabase.html). Point mutations account for the majority of mutations (~90%) and large exon deletion mutations account for ~6%. Complex rearrangement mutations without exonal dosage changes (copy-neutral) have rarely been reported; large inversion mutations such as intron 22 inversion in HA have not been reported in HB. Missense/nonsense mutations account for ~70% of point mutations, followed by small insertion/deletion mutations (~17%). In addition, it is notable that whole gene deletions account for approximately half of the large exon deletion mutations in *F9*. Based on the line of evidence collected from the literature and mutation database, the following is a proposed procedure for profiling *F9* mutations (Figure 7).

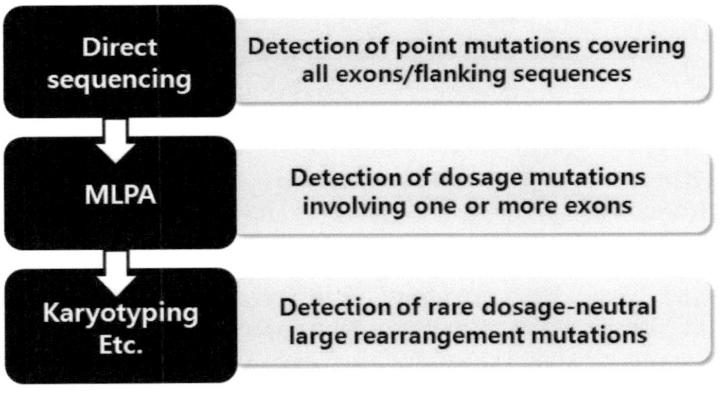

Fig. 7. A proposed strategy of *F9* mutation profiling.

3.1 Identification of *F9* point mutations by direct sequencing analysis

As point mutations account for ~90% of cases, direct sequencing can be the first-line diagnostic modality for molecular diagnosis in HB. As in HA, the mutations are scattered throughout the gene, thus, sequencing analyses need to cover the coding sequences and flanking intronic sequences of all 8 exons (Kwon et al., 2008). The strategy for direct sequencing analysis is largely similar to that for HA, but is simpler and less costly because the *F9* gene is smaller and is encoded by a smaller number of exons. In addition, as in HA, mutation scanning by CSGE can also be applied for direct sequencing analyses, but the detection sensitivity of CSGE needs to be validated in each laboratory prior to clinical implementation (Santacroce et al., 2008). Large deletion mutations, which can be detected by MLPA analyses, should be suspected when 1 or more reactions to amplify a genomic segment fail. Below is an example of a sequencing result with a missense mutation in a Korean HB (Kwon et al., 2008).

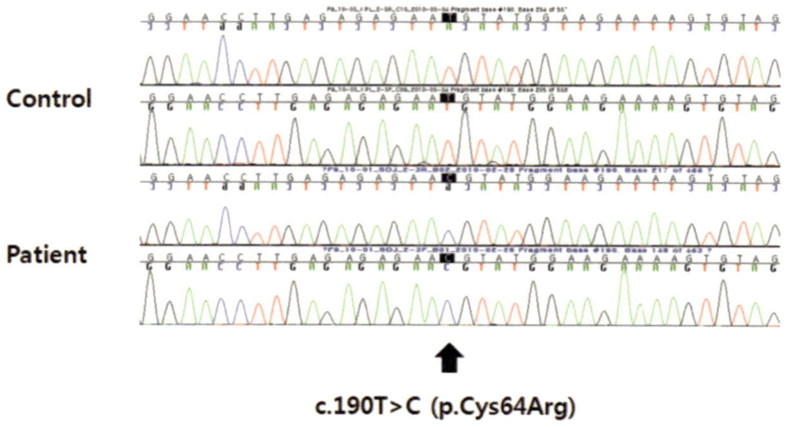

Fig. 8. A point mutation (missense mutation) leading to the substituion of the 64th amino acid residue cysteine to arginine detected by direct sequencing analyses in a Korean male patient with HB

3.2 Identification of large exon deletion mutations by multiplex ligation-dependent probe amplification

The possibility of large exon deletion mutations should be considered (second-line molecular genetic test in HB) when no point mutations are identified through direct sequencing analyses or when PCR experiments fail on 1 or more exons. As in HA, the MLPA technique is a robust molecular test to detect mutations of large exon deletion affecting 1 or more exons in *F9* (Kwon et al., 2008). The principle and method of interpretation of MLPA results are similar to that for *F8*. The detection of this type of mutation is particularly important since it implicates a high risk of inhibitor development (Giannelli et al., 1983; Oldenburg et al., 2004). The real-time quantitative PCR technique can also be used to detect large exon deletion mutations in *F9* (Vencesla et al., 2007). However, recent studies have pointed out the advantages of MLPA over real-time PCR (Casana et al., 2009). Figure 9 is an example of a result of a multiplex ligation-dependent probe amplification experiment with whole gene deletion in a Korean male HB.

3.3 Identification of large rearrangement mutations without large exon deletion changes

The need to search for copy-neutral large rearrangement mutations arises when no point mutations or large exon deletion mutations are detected on direct sequencing followed by MLPA analyses. In particular, a balanced chromosomal rearrangement involving the *F9* gene on the Xq27.1 band disrupts the normal transcription and translation of the molecule, leading to HB. Karyotype analyses using peripheral blood lymphocytes can detect rearrangements such as t(X;1)(q27.1;q22 or q23) and t(X;15)(q27.1;p11.2) (Ghosh et al., 2009; Schroder, W. et al., 1998). In particular, these rearrangements can be the genetic backgrounds of female HB with or without family history. X chromosome analyses are needed in such cases to confirm skewed inactivation of the non-rearranged copy of the X chromosome.

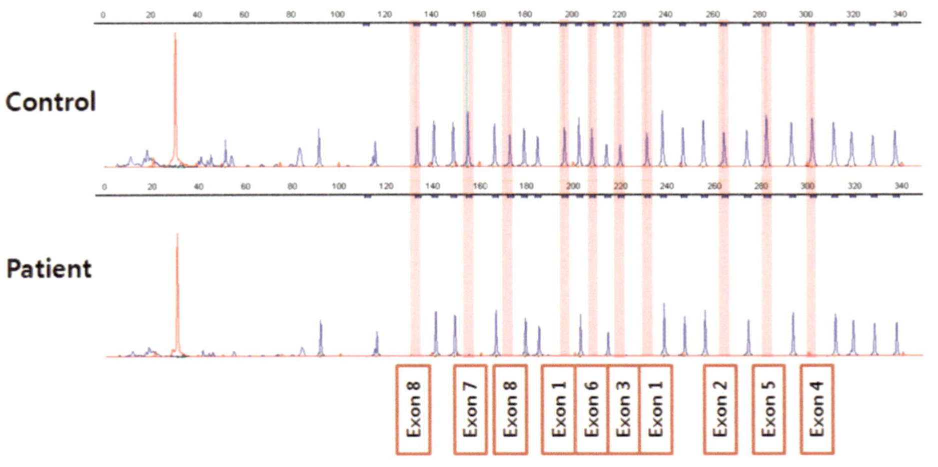

Fig. 9. The chromatographic results of the multiplex ligation-dependent probe amplificaiton experiment showing the whole *F9* gene deletion in a male patient with haemophilia B

4. New approach of the mutation profiling

Technologies for more efficient detection of mutations such as microarrays and next generation sequencing (NGS) have been developed. Although mutation testing with microarrays has received attention, it faces limitations in identifying various mutations (Berber et al., 2006; Chan et al., 2005). In addition, microarray-identified mutations require validation to eliminate false positive or false negative results (Johnson et al., 2010). On that point, NGS is a prospective approach in *F8* mutation studies (Lindblom & Robinson, 2011). NGS is an alternative sequencing strategy that redefines "high-throughput sequencing". These technologies outperform the older Sanger-based sequencing by throughput capacity and reduce the cost of sequencing. However, NGS still faces some problems in application to *F8* or *F9* sequencing for mutation identification. The cost of NGS equipment is more expensive than that of other capillary sequencing machines. As NGS sifts through a large amount of data, a bioinformatics expert is needed to analyze the high-throughput sequencing data. Recently, NGS companies have begun launching mini-scale (personal sequencing system) equipment.

Typical examples of mini-scale NGS machines are the GS junior system from Roche, which is based on 454 sequencing, the MiSeq from Illumina, and the Ion torrent from Life Technology. These equipments can amplify 10–100 M genes with proven technology (Glenn, 2011). Moreover, they can be applied variously to amplicon sequencing assays, small genome sequencing, exome sequencing, and genome-wide association study (GWAS) targeted regions (Grossmann et al., 2011). They also require neither bulky equipments for analysis nor lengthy time to produce a large amount of results. These advantages of mini-scale sequencing are considered useful for the identification of *F8* or *F9* sequence variants. Established capillary electrophoresis requires at least 40 reactions to analyze the 26 exons in the *F8* gene from 1 person. It would take approximately 3,840 sequencing reactions to survey 96 patients for the *F8* mutation (Grossmann et al., 2011). This uses a lot of money and

is labor intensive. However, the MiSeq system and TruSeq® amplicon sequencing method requires just 1 sequencing reaction to carry out the task and a week to analyze *F8* sequence variations. This prospective tool could be widely used in hemophilia diagnosis.

5. Concluding comments

Mutations in *F8* result in truncated FVIII proteins, which can affect their interaction with other proteins in the coagulation cascade. Some mutations affect the recognition region of molecular chaperone proteins in the Golgi apparatus or endoplasmic reticulum during post-translational modification of FVIII (Dorner et al., 1987; Lenting et al., 1998; Leyte et al., 1991). Another consideration of the *F8* or *F9* mutation is closely related with the development of inhibitory antibodies. For these reasons, effective profiling of mutations in *F8* or *F9* is important for the diagnosis and therapy of hemophilia, as well as prediction of inhibitor development.

6. References

Bagnall, R.D., Waseem, N., Green, P.M., & Giannelli, F. (2002), Recurrent inversion breaking intron 1 of the factor VIII gene is a frequent cause of severe hemophilia A, *Blood*, Vol. 99, No. 1, pp 168-174, ISSN 0006-4971 (Print).

Berber, E., Leggo, J., Brown, C., Gallo, N., Feilotter, H., & Lillicrap, D. (2006), DNA microarray analysis for the detection of mutations in hemophilia A, *J Thromb Haemost*, Vol. 4, No. 8, pp 1756-1762, ISSN 1538-7933 (Print), 1538-7836 (Linking).

Boekhorst, J., Lari, G.R., D'Oiron, R., Costa, J.M., Novakova, I.R., Ala, F.A., Lavergne, J.M., & WL, V.A.N.H. (2008), Factor VIII genotype and inhibitor development in patients with haemophilia A: highest risk in patients with splice site mutations, *Haemophilia*, Vol. 14, No. 4, pp 729-735, ISSN 1365-2516 (Electronic), 1351-8216 (Linking).

Bogdanova, N., Markoff, A., Pollmann, H., Nowak-Gottl, U., Eisert, R., Wermes, C., Todorova, A., Eigel, A., Dworniczak, B., & Horst, J. (2005), Spectrum of molecular defects and mutation detection rate in patients with severe hemophilia A, *Hum Mutat*, Vol. 26, No. 3, pp 249-254, ISSN 1098-1004 (Electronic), 1059-7794 (Linking).

Bowen, D.J. (2002), Haemophilia A and haemophilia B: molecular insights, *Mol Pathol*, Vol. 55, No. 1, pp 1-18, ISSN 1366-8714 (Print).

Casana, P., Haya, S., Cid, A.R., Oltra, S., Martinez, F., Cabrera, N., & Aznar, J.A. (2009), Identification of deletion carriers in hemophilia B: quantitative real-time polymerase chain reaction or multiple ligation probe amplification, *Transl Res*, Vol. 153, No. 3, pp 114-117, ISSN 1931-5244 (Print), 1878-1810 (Linking).

Chan, K., Sasanakul, W., Mellars, G., Chuansumrit, A., Perry, D., Lee, C.A., Wong, M.S., Chan, T.K., & Chan, V. (2005), Detection of known haemophilia B mutations and carrier testing by microarray, *Thromb Haemost*, Vol. 94, No. 4, pp 872-878, ISSN 0340-6245 (Print), 0340-6245 (Linking).

Chao, H., Mansfield, S.G., Bartel, R.C., Hiriyanna, S., Mitchell, L.G., Garcia-Blanco, M.A., & Walsh, C.E. (2003), Phenotype correction of hemophilia A mice by spliceosome-mediated RNA trans-splicing, *Nat Med*, Vol. 9, No. 8, pp 1015-1019, ISSN 1078-8956 (Print), 1078-8956 (Linking).

David, D., et al. (1994), Analysis of the essential sequences of the factor VIII gene in twelve haemophilia A patients by single-stranded conformation polymorphism, *Blood Coagul Fibrinolysis*, Vol. 5, No. 2, pp 257-264, ISSN 0957-5235 (Print), 0957-5235 (Linking).

Di Scipio, R.G., Kurachi, K., & Davie, E.W. (1978), Activation of human factor IX (Christmas factor), *J Clin Invest*, Vol. 61, No. 6, pp 1528-1538, ISSN 0021-9738 (Print), 0021-9738 (Linking).

Dorner, A.J., Bole, D.G., & Kaufman, R.J. (1987), The relationship of N-linked glycosylation and heavy chain-binding protein association with the secretion of glycoproteins, *J Cell Biol*, Vol. 105, No. 6 Pt 1, pp 2665-2674, ISSN 0021-9525 (Print).

El-Maarri, O., et al. (2005), Analysis of mRNA in hemophilia A patients with undetectable mutations reveals normal splicing in the factor VIII gene, *J Thromb Haemost*, Vol. 3, No. 2, pp 332-339, ISSN 1538-7933 (Print), 1538-7836 (Linking).

Fidanci, I.D., Kavakli, K., Ucar, C., Timur, C., Meral, A., Kilinc, Y., Sayilan, H., Kazanci, E., & Caglayan, S.H. (2008), Factor 8 (F8) gene mutation profile of Turkish hemophilia A patients with inhibitors, *Blood Coagul Fibrinolysis*, Vol. 19, No. 5, pp 383-388, ISSN 0957-5235 (Print), 0957-5235 (Linking).

Ghosh, K., Shetty, S., Quadros, L., & Kulkarni, B. (2009), Double mutations causing haemophilia B: a double whammy!, *Br J Haematol*, Vol. 145, No. 3, pp 433-435, ISSN 1365-2141 (Electronic), 0007-1048 (Linking).

Giannelli, F., Choo, K.H., Rees, D.J., Boyd, Y., Rizza, C.R., & Brownlee, G.G. (1983), Gene deletions in patients with haemophilia B and anti-factor IX antibodies, *Nature*, Vol. 303, No. 5913, pp 181-182, ISSN 0028-0836 (Print), 0028-0836 (Linking).

Glenn, T.C. (2011), Field guide to next-generation DNA sequencers, *Mol Ecol Resour*, ISSN 1755-0998 (Electronic), 1755-098X (Linking).

Graw, J., Brackmann, H.H., Oldenburg, J., Schneppenheim, R., Spannagl, M., & Schwaab, R. (2005), Haemophilia A: from mutation analysis to new therapies, *Nat Rev Genet*, Vol. 6, No. 6, pp 488-501, ISSN 1471-0056 (Print).

Grossmann, V., Kohlmann, A., Klein, H.U., Schindela, S., Schnittger, S., Dicker, F., Dugas, M., Kern, W., Haferlach, T., & Haferlach, C. (2011), Targeted next-generation sequencing detects point mutations, insertions, deletions and balanced chromosomal rearrangements as well as identifies novel leukemia-specific fusion genes in a single procedure, *Leukemia*, Vol. 25, No. 4, pp 671-680, ISSN 1476-5551 (Electronic), 0887-6924 (Linking).

Hwang, S.H., Kim, M.J., Lim, J.A., Kim, H.C., & Kim, H.S. (2009), Profiling of factor VIII mutations in Korean haemophilia A, *Haemophilia*, Vol. 15, No. 6, pp 1311-1317, ISSN 1365-2516 (Electronic), 1351-8216 (Linking).

Johnson, D.S., et al. (2010), Preclinical validation of a microarray method for full molecular karyotyping of blastomeres in a 24-h protocol, *Hum Reprod*, Vol. 25, No. 4, pp 1066-1075, ISSN 1460-2350 (Electronic), 0268-1161 (Linking).

Korkko, J., Annunen, S., Pihlajamaa, T., Prockop, D.J., & Ala-Kokko, L. (1998), Conformation sensitive gel electrophoresis for simple and accurate detection of mutations: comparison with denaturing gradient gel electrophoresis and nucleotide sequencing, *Proc Natl Acad Sci U S A*, Vol. 95, No. 4, pp 1681-1685, ISSN 0027-8424 (Print), 0027-8424 (Linking).

Kwon, M.J., Yoo, K.Y., Kim, H.J., & Kim, S.H. (2008), Identification of mutations in the F9 gene including exon deletion by multiplex ligation-dependent probe amplification in 33 unrelated Korean patients with haemophilia B, *Haemophilia,* Vol. 14, No. 5, pp 1069-1075, ISSN 1365-2516 (Electronic), 1351-8216 (Linking).

Lannoy, N., Abinet, I., Dahan, K., & Hermans, C. (2009), Identification of de novo deletion in the factor VIII gene by MLPA technique in two girls with isolated factor VIII deficiency, *Haemophilia,* Vol. 15, No. 3, pp 797-801, ISSN 1365-2516 (Electronic), 1351-8216 (Linking).

Lenting, P.J., van Mourik, J.A., & Mertens, K. (1998), The life cycle of coagulation factor VIII in view of its structure and function, *Blood,* Vol. 92, No. 11, pp 3983-3996, ISSN 0006-4971 (Print).

Leyte, A., van Schijndel, H.B., Niehrs, C., Huttner, W.B., Verbeet, M.P., Mertens, K., & van Mourik, J.A. (1991), Sulfation of Tyr1680 of human blood coagulation factor VIII is essential for the interaction of factor VIII with von Willebrand factor, *J Biol Chem,* Vol. 266, No. 2, pp 740-746, ISSN 0021-9258 (Print),

Lindblom, A., & Robinson, P.N. (2011), Bioinformatics for human genetics: promises and challenges, *Hum Mutat,* Vol. 32, No. 5, pp 495-500, ISSN 1098-1004 (Electronic), 1059-7794 (Linking).

Lindquist, P.A., Fujikawa, K., & Davie, E.W. (1978), Activation of bovine factor IX (Christmas factor) by factor XIa (activated plasma thromboplastin antecedent) and a protease from Russell's viper venom, *J Biol Chem,* Vol. 253, No. 6, pp 1902-1909, ISSN 0021-9258 (Print), 0021-9258 (Linking).

Liu, Q., Nozari, G., & Sommer, S.S. (1998), Single-tube polymerase chain reaction for rapid diagnosis of the inversion hotspot of mutation in hemophilia A, *Blood,* Vol. 92, No. 4, pp 1458-1459, ISSN 0006-4971 (Print), 0006-4971 (Linking).

Mahajan, A., Chavali, S., Ghosh, S., Kabra, M., Chowdhury, M.R., & Bharadwaj, D. (2007), Allelic heterogeneity of molecular events in human coagulation factor IX in Asian Indians. Mutation in brief #965. Online, *Hum Mutat,* Vol. 28, No. 5, pp 526, ISSN 1098-1004 (Electronic), 1059-7794 (Linking).

Oldenburg, J., Brackmann, H.H., & Schwaab, R. (2000), Risk factors for inhibitor development in hemophilia A, *Haematologica,* Vol. 85, No. 10 Suppl, pp 7-13; discussion 13-14, ISSN 0390-6078 (Print), 0390-6078 (Linking).

Oldenburg, J., El-Maarri, O., & Schwaab, R. (2002), Inhibitor development in correlation to factor VIII genotypes, *Haemophilia,* Vol. 8 Suppl 2, pp 23-29, ISSN 1351-8216 (Print), 1351-8216 (Linking).

Oldenburg, J., Schroder, J., Brackmann, H.H., Muller-Reible, C., Schwaab, R., & Tuddenham, E. (2004), Environmental and genetic factors influencing inhibitor development, *Semin Hematol,* Vol. 41, No. 1 Suppl 1, pp 82-88, ISSN 0037-1963 (Print), 0037-1963 (Linking).

Polakova, H., Zmetakova, I., & Kadasi, L. (2003), Long distance PCR in detection of inversion mutations of F8C gene in hemophilia A patients, *Gen Physiol Biophys,* Vol. 22, No. 2, pp 243-253, ISSN 0231-5882 (Print).

Repesse, Y., Slaoui, M., Ferrandiz, D., Gautier, P., Costa, C., Costa, J.M., Lavergne, J.M., & Borel-Derlon, A. (2007), Factor VIII (FVIII) gene mutations in 120 patients with hemophilia A: detection of 26 novel mutations and correlation with FVIII inhibitor

development, *J Thromb Haemost*, Vol. 5, No. 7, pp 1469-1476, ISSN 1538-7933 (Print), 1538-7836 (Linking).

Santacroce, R., et al. (2008), Identification of 217 unreported mutations in the F8 gene in a group of 1,410 unselected Italian patients with hemophilia A, *J Hum Genet*, Vol. 53, No. 3, pp 275-284, ISSN 1434-5161 (Print), 1434-5161 (Linking).

Schroder, J., El-Maarri, O., Schwaab, R., Muller, C.R., & Oldenburg, J. (2006), Factor VIII intron-1 inversion: frequency and inhibitor prevalence, *J Thromb Haemost*, Vol. 4, No. 5, pp 1141-1143, ISSN 1538-7933 (Print), 1538-7836 (Linking).

Schroder, W., Poetsch, M., Gazda, H., Werner, W., Reichelt, T., Knoll, W., Rokicka-Milewska, R., Zieleniewska, B., & Herrmann, F.H. (1998), A de novo translocation 46,X,t(X;15) causing haemophilia B in a girl: a case report, *Br J Haematol*, Vol. 100, No. 4, pp 750-757, ISSN 0007-1048 (Print), 0007-1048 (Linking).

Tagariello, G., Belvini, D., Salviato, R., Di Gaetano, R., Zanotto, D., Radossi, P., Risato, R., Sartori, R., & Tassinari, C. (2007), The Italian haemophilia B mutation database: a tool for genetic counselling, carrier detection and prenatal diagnosis, *Blood Transfus*, Vol. 5, No. 3, pp 158-163, ISSN 1723-2007 (Print), 1723-2007 (Linking).

Tuddenham, E.G., et al. (1994), Haemophilia A: database of nucleotide substitutions, deletions, insertions and rearrangements of the factor VIII gene, second edition, *Nucleic Acids Res*, Vol. 22, No. 17, pp 3511-3533, ISSN 0305-1048 (Print), 0305-1048 (Linking).

Vencesla, A., Barcelo, M.J., Baena, M., Quintana, M., Baiget, M., & Tizzano, E.F. (2007), Marker and real-time quantitative analyses to confirm hemophilia B carrier diagnosis of a complete deletion of the F9 gene, *Haematologica*, Vol. 92, No. 11, pp 1583-1584, ISSN 1592-8721 (Electronic), 0390-6078 (Linking).

Yoshitake, S., Schach, B.G., Foster, D.C., Davie, E.W., & Kurachi, K. (1985), Nucleotide sequence of the gene for human factor IX (antihemophilic factor B), *Biochemistry*, Vol. 24, No. 14, pp 3736-3750, ISSN 0006-2960 (Print), 0006-2960 (Linking).

2

Genotype-Phenotype Interaction Analyses in Hemophilia

Ana Rebeca Jaloma-Cruz et al.*
División de Genética, Centro de Investigación Biomédica de Occidente
Instituto Mexicano del Seguro Social
México

1. Introduction

As with monogenic diseases, hemophilia A and hemophilia B have a direct relationship between factor VIII and factor IX gene mutations, respectively, and their causative effect on protein deficiency either in function or reduced antigen level in plasma. These aspects are related to, but do not totally explain, a more complex clinical phenotype such as the age of initial symptom onset, bleeding tendency, inhibitor development, arthropathy tendency, carrier bleeding symptoms, etc., which currently are critical complications under study in various clinical protocols in order to improve medical care in patients with hemophilia.

The complex relationship between clinical behavior and genetics of hemophilia is changing the approach to diagnosis and research methods, expanding the scope of analysis to other related genes (bleeding tendency, immune system, regulatory genes of X-chromosome expression, etc.). In addition, novel functional approaches can provide prognostic parameters of clinical behavior such as gene expression assays and biochemical analyses including kinetics of inhibitors to factor VIII or thrombin generation assay by the standardized method of calibrated automated thrombography. This method describes the overall clotting capacity of patients' plasma *in vitro* and *ex vivo*. This chapter will focus on certain studies regarding genotype-phenotype interactions in hemophilia that have been applied in Mexican hemophilia families for molecular diagnosis and genetic counseling. These studies have also been used to determine prognostic factors for clinical behavior and treatment response in hemophilia patients in order to improve hematological management as well as to optimize the use of therapeutic resources, an important consideration in developing countries such as Mexico.

* Claudia Patricia Beltrán-Miranda, Isaura Araceli González-Ramos, José de Jesús López-Jiménez, Hilda Luna-Záizar, Johanna Milena Mantilla-Capacho, Jessica Noemi Mundo-Ayala and Mayra Judith Valdés Galván
División de Genética, Centro de Investigación Biomédica de Occidente
Instituto Mexicano del Seguro Social
México

2. Mutation–phenotype correlation in hemophilia

2.1 Origin of mutations in hemophilia

Because of the high mutation rate of *factor VIII* gene (2.5–4.2 x 10^{5}), ~50% of the severely affected families have only one affected case (isolated), pointing to a recent mutation occurring in the grandparental or parental generation. Family studies reveal that most mutations in hemophilia A originate in male germ cells with a predominance of point mutations. Some deletions occur in female gametes and *de novo* mutations may occur in early embryogenesis from a somatic or germinal mosaicism. This mechanism, if minor, remains underestimated by routine analysis and originates predominantly from females in the case of somatic mosaicism. This may represent a frequent event in hemophilia that must be considered in genetic counseling of isolated cases that mainly involve point mutations (Leuer et al., 2001).

In the case of *factor IX* gene, a considerably lower mutation rate than for *factor VIII* has been reported (3.2 x 10^{9}) (Koeberl et al., 1990). However, in hemophilia B there is also a high proportion of recent germline mutations originating in the last three generations of isolated cases that have been studied in different populations. A similar mutation pattern has been found, suggesting an endogenous mechanism for the genetic changes in *factor IX* gene causing hemophilia B. The endogenous mechanism indicates that genetic characteristics of the gene (rather than environmental conditions) account for most human germline mutations (Sommer 1995, as cited in Jaloma-Cruz et al., 2000). Point mutations are the most common mutations in hemophilia, being present in >90% of the patients. This is followed by deletions in 5-10% of the cases. Less frequent are the insertion/inversion rearrangements with the exception of intron 22 inversion of *factor VIII* gene in hemophilia A. This is the most common genetic rearrangement demonstrated in severe disease, comprising 40-50% of cases (Bowen, 2002).

2.2 Mutation pattern in hemophilia

There is a high degree of heterogeneity in the location and type of mutations in *factor VIII* and *factor IX* genes causing hemophilia; >90% are located in coding and promoter regions as well in junction sites of intron-exon. Types of mutation and their relative frequencies are determined by genetic mechanisms according to the genetic sequence (mutation hot-spots such as CpG dinucleotides, gene size, nucleotide repeats, etc.). A general pattern of mutations is found as follows: single nucleotide changes: transitions > transversions; deletions > insertions > complex rearrangements (Sommer, 1995, as cited in Jaloma-Cruz et al., 2000).

2.3 Unusual mutagenesis mechanism in the Mexican hemophilia B population

From a study of nine independent Mexican hemophilia B families (Jaloma-Cruz et al., 2000), we found a particular mechanism of recurrent mutagenesis by four single independent substitutions in two similar non-CpG sites at nucleotide positions 17,678 (C88Y, C88F) and 17,747 (C111S, C111Y) of *factor IX* gene (Table 1). Using a statistical test considering a mutation target of 439 nucleotide position non-CpG sites in the coding region of *factor IX* (where >96% of *factor IX* gene mutations occur), it was demonstrated that the observed mutations were nonrandom events ($p = 0.0004$) (Jaloma-Cruz et al., 2000). These mutations were considered as first-line evidence of a mechanism of recurrent mutation in hemophilia involving unusual hot-spot sites. It will be interesting to continue these types of studies in

epidemiological analyses to explore the subjacent mechanism of causative mutagenesis in particular populations.

Proband (Clinical)[a]	Mutation	Effect	Origin[b]	Geographical Region	Haplotype[c]
HB 758 (M)	17747G>C	C111S	Familial	Michoacan, Central Pacific Coast	C/-/I/-/-/IV/-
HB 759 (S)	Exons F,G&H	LD[d]	Familial	Michoacan, Central Pacific Coast	C/-/I/-/-/
HB 760 (M)	17678G>A	C88Y	*de novo* MF	Jalisco, Central Pacific Coast	T/-/I/-/-/IV/-
HB 762 (S)	20519G>A@CpG	R180Q	*de novo* MM	Nuevo Leon, Northeast	C/-/I/-/-/II/-
HB 763 (M)	31284-5del AG	fs[e]	Familial	Michoacan, Central Pacific Coast	C/-/I/-/-/II/+
HB 764 (S)	20519G>A@CpG	R180Q	Sporadic	Sinaloa, North Pacific Coast	C/-/I/-/-/II/-
HB 765 (M)	17747G>A	C111Y	*de novo* M	Nuevo Leon, Northeast	C/-/I/-/-/II/-
HB 766 (S)	Exons G&H	LD[d]	Familial	Michoacan, Central Pacific Coast	C/-/I/+/+/
HB 767 (N)	17678G>T	C88F	Sporadic	Puebla, Central	C/-/I/-/-/II/+

Table 1. Summary of Mutations in Mexican Patients with Hemophilia B

[a]S = Severe; M = Moderate; N = No data (White, 2001).
[b]HB760: the sequence change at 17678 was present in the index patient and mother, but absent from both maternal grandmother and grandfather. The 3'RY(i) polymorphism, established the maternal grandfather (MF) as the origin. HB762: the mother was a carrier, but the sequence change at 20,519 was not present in 13 maternal aunts and uncles or in the maternal grandfather. Extragenic polymorphisms, *DXS 1211* and *DXS 1232*, established the maternal grandmother (MM) as the origin.
HB765: the sequence change at 17,747 was present only in the index patient, establishing the mother (M) as the origin.
[c]*Mse*I/*BamHI*/*Hinf*I/*Xmn*I/*Taq*I/3'RY(i)/*Hha*I.
[d]LD, large deletions. The *MCF2* gene, located about 80 kb downstream of the *F9* transcription start site is present in HB759 but absent in HB766, indicating deletions of about 60 kb and more than 100 kb, respectively.
[e]Microdeletion resulting in frameshift (fs) at G388 and stop codon at I408.
(Modified from Jaloma et al., 2000)

2.4 Genotype-phenotype correlation in hemophilia

As with monogenic diseases, hemophilia A and B have a direct relationship between *factor VIII* and *factor IX* gene mutations, respectively, and their causative phenotype effect at the clinical level secondary to the caused protein deficiency, either in function or reduced antigen level in plasma (Koeberl et al., 1990).

In general, there is good correlation between the type of mutation (location in the amino-acid position and domain in the protein) and their functional outcome, yielding a predictable clinical severity. However, some authors affirm that this correlation is rare and, in the majority of cases, a clear correlation has not been shown (Bowen, 2002) with the exception in a very few cases of self-evident molecular defects such as large deletions,

nonsense mutations causing premature translation stop and truncated protein, corrupted mRNA splicing, etc.
Because of the difficulty in presenting a clear correlation, in 2001 the International Committee of Standardization in Thrombosis and Hemostasis established the clinical severity classification according to the clotting level in plasma and not to clinical manifestations (more complex phenotype). A direct relationship between the genetic defect and protein activity is expected (Table 2) (White, 2001).

Factor Level	Classification
< 0.01 IU/ml (<1% of normal)	Severe
0.01 – 0.05 IU/ml (1%-5% of normal)	Moderate
> 0.05 - < 0.40 IU/ml (>5% - <40% of normal)	Mild

Table 2. Classification of hemophilia A and B. Normal is 1 IU/ml of factor VIII:C (valid also for factor IX:C) as defined by the current World Health Organization International Standard for Plasma Factor VIII:C (as distributed by The National Institute for Biological Standards and Control, Potters Bar, Hertsfordshire, UK). *(Modified from White et al., 2001).*

The limitation of the criterion of clotting activity of deficient factors VIII and IX to establish clinical severity in hemophilia may be due to the fault of reproducibility of laboratory tests of coagulation. These may be due to assay problems such as sample management (preanalytical factors), quality of reagents, zero point activity, etc., that must be carefully controlled in order to have a confident result and the relationship with clinical severity (Barrowcliffe, 2004). These problems also lead to investigation of newer methods with closer physiological correlation, higher sensitivity and less coefficient variation values such as thrombin generation test or thromboelastography (Barrowcliffe, 2004).

3. Structure-function relationship of *factor IX* gene mutations at the subcellular level

During the search for mechanisms that cause mutations in hemophilia and its impact on the relationship between the structure-function of mutant proteins, several analytical investigations have been developed at the cellular level of the interaction of factor VIII (FVIII) and factor IX (FIX) mutant proteins with other intracellular components involved in their posttranslational processing and secretion.

3.1 Structure-function relationship in mutant FIX proteins

In the study of *factor IX* mutations causing a severe phenotype, two mutations were analysed. These were located at the first and second epidermal growth factor (EGF) domain,

C71Y and C109Y, respectively, both affecting a cysteine site and, therefore, the folding native structure of FIX protein (Enjolras et al., 2004). Different analyses of posttranslational processing and intracellular trafficking revealed that neither mutant was secreted nor accumulated in the intracellular space due to their interaction with chaperones from endoplasmic reticulum (ER) that cause their arrest and lead to their degradation into proteasomes (Enjolras et al., 2004). A related study was carried out for the relevant *factor IX* mutations identified in Mexican hemophilia B patients that were caused by a recurrent mutagenesis at non-CpG sites (Jaloma-Cruz et al., 2000). They also affected the structure-function of FIX by changes of a cysteine position in the second epidermal growth factor (EGF2) domain of *factor IX* gene (C111S and C111Y mutations).

3.2 Directed mutagenesis and functional analysis of FIX mutations

The two mutations at cysteine 111 cause severe hemophilia B in Mexican hemophilia B patients. To analyze their impact on the structure-function relationship of FIX, the effect of inhibitors of intracellular trafficking was studied comparing C111 wild-type (wt) and the C111S and C111Y mutations that were inserted by directed-site mutagenesis into an expression vector (pcDNA 3.1®) containing *factor IX* wild type (wt) gene. Transfection by Fugene6® was evaluated in Cos-7 cells after 48 h. Intracellular production and secretion of FIX were quantified by ELISA assay. Transfected cells were incubated for 6 h with different inhibitors of intracellular trafficking classified by their solubility properties; hydrosolubles: NH_4Cl and leupeptin, which are lysosomal inhibitors, and liposolubles: Brefeldin A, that blocks protein transport from ER to the Golgi complex; cycloheximide, inhibitor of synthesis protein, N-acetyl-leu-leu-norleucinal (ALLN) and clasto-lactacystin beta-lactone (calpain), both proteasomal inhibitors (Mantilla-Capacho et al., 2008).

The mutants showed a decreased FIX secretion (20%) and intracellular accumulation of 140% (C111Y) and 160% (C111S) with respect to wt *factor IX*. The inhibitors caused higher intracellular accumulation, which evidenced a degradation primarily in lysosomes (NH_4Cl) of both mutants. C111S mutation showed a strong effect of Brefeldin A, suggesting an adequate transport from ER to Golgi complex in contrast to C111Y, which showed higher proteasomal degradation, evidenced by the effect of ALLN (Figure 1) (Mantilla-Capacho et al., 2008).

The study concluded that the disruption of the disulfide bond in the mutants has an important effect on the native folding of FIX due to their accumulation in the intracellular space in regard to wt FIX. C111Y showed a higher impact than C111S on its transport through ER with a predominant degradation at proteasomes (Mantilla-Capacho et al., 2008).

Other *factor IX* mutations previously identified in the Mexican population have also been analyzed using related approaches for the analysis of genotype-phenotype interaction at the subcellular level. These demonstrate evidence of posttranscriptional regulation mechanisms and behavior of mutant proteins that reveal the importance of key sites of protein function. Further studies are essential for a better understanding of the properties of FVIII and FIX and the biochemical phenotype of hemophilia.

4. Molecular diagnosis for carrier testing

The wide mutational heterogeneity in both types of hemophilia compels the use of intragenic polymorphisms for carrier testing. Different polymorphisms have been described in *factor VIII* and *factor IX* genes such as single nucleotide polymorphisms (SNPs) identified

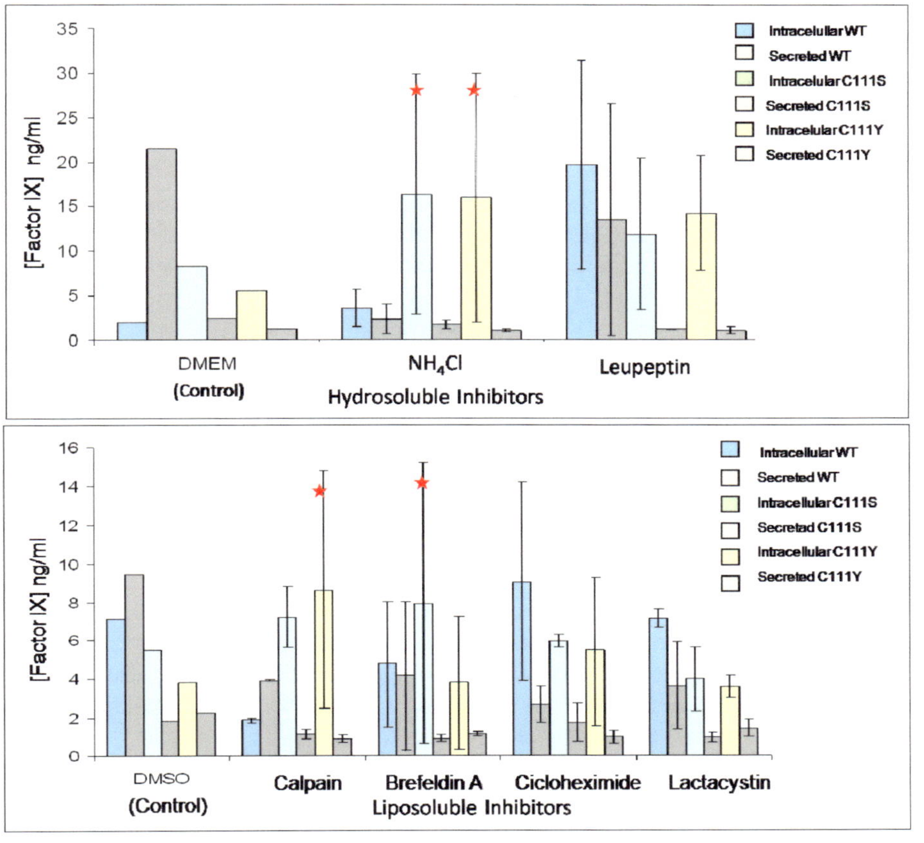

Fig. 1. Effect of inhibitors of cellular trafficking on factor IX production (intracellular and secretion) of C111S and C111Y mutations of *factor IX* gene. Significant effect is highlighted by red stars.

by restriction fragment length enzyme polymorphisms (RFLPs), variable number of tandem repeats (VNTRs) or microsatellites defined by the length of the repeated units [1-4 nucleotides, short tandem repeats (STRs), >5 nucleotides, VNTRs] (Bowen, 2002). According to recent knowledge of the human genome and the high variability among individuals, a difference is expected of one base for every 1250 base pairs on average. According to the gene sizes of *factor VIII* (186 kb) and *factor IX* (34 kb), both genes would be expected to be ~144 and 27 SNPs, respectively. However, fewer polymorphisms have been identified, which means a paucity of polymorphisms or a detection problem, this last reason being more plausible because new polymorphisms continue to be described (Figure 2) (Bowen, 2002; Kim, 2005).

4.1 Linkage analysis in hemophilia A and B

Automatic sequencing methods and high-yield analysis techniques of the human genome have extended the detection of mutations in both types of hemophilias. In the case of *factor VIII* and *factor IX* genes, diverse polymorphisms have been used for carrier diagnosis as a low cost, alternative and rapid method. Use of intragenic polymorphisms by linkage analysis shows high confidence (>95%) according to the linkage disequilibrium between

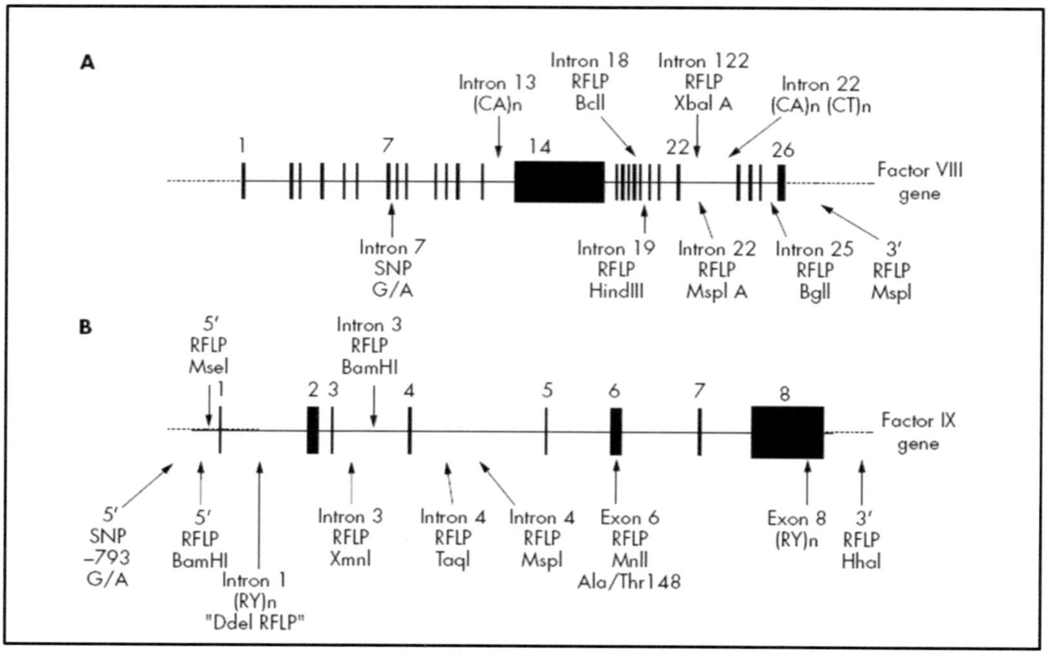

Fig. 2. Polymorphisms of *factor VIII* and *factor IX* genes. Some of the known polymorphisms in the human genes for (A) factor VIII and (B) factor IX.

a) Factor VIII gene: intron 7 G/A, intron 13 (CA)n, intron 18 *Bcl*I, intron 19 *Hind*III, intron 22 *Xba*I A, intron 22 *Msp*I A, intron 22 (CA)n, intron 25 *Bgl*I, 3'*Msp*I.
b) Factor IX gene: 5' -793 G/A, 5' *Bam*HI, 5' *Mse*I, intron 1 *Dde*I, intron 3 *Xmn*I, intron 3 *Bam*HI, intron 4 *Taq*I, intron 4 *Msp*I, exon 6 *Mnl*I, exon 8 (RY)n, and 3' *Hha*I.
(Figure and source references of polymorphisms as cited in Bowen, 2002).

polymorphisms and the causative mutation of the hemophilia (Mantilla-Capacho et al., 2005). This strategy requires sampling of all family members to trace the segregation of the polymorphism linked to the mutated X-chromosome for *factor VIII* or *factor IX* genes. The main limitation of the strategy is the informativeness of the polymorphism that is defined by its heterozygosity in a population, with a maximum value of 50%, corresponding to the highest probability of finding two alleles in the obligated carrier of one family. The described polymorphisms must be analyzed in each population in order to identify the useful markers.

4.2 Carrier diagnosis strategy in the Mexican population

For molecular analysis of carrier diagnosis, we developed a strategy based on intragenic polymorphism linkage analysis. According to their diagnostic informativeness percentage in the Mexican population, for *factor VIII* gene we initially used the following: the microsatellite of (CA)n of intron 13 (75%) and the RFLPs *Bcl*I- intron 18 (50%) and *Alw*NI-intron 7 (20%) (Mantilla-Capacho et al., 2005).
In order to improve the technical feasibility and informative level of carrier diagnosis in Mexican families with hemophilia A, we used the method of Kim et al. (2005) based on fluorescent PCR of four intragenic dinucleotide-repeat polymorphisms analyzed by automated Genescan®. Preliminary data show that the use of dinucleotide repeats at introns

1, 13 and 22 achieved a significant increase in informativeness (>85%), which is useful for carrier testing in more than 200 hemophilia A families (González-Ramos et al., 2010).

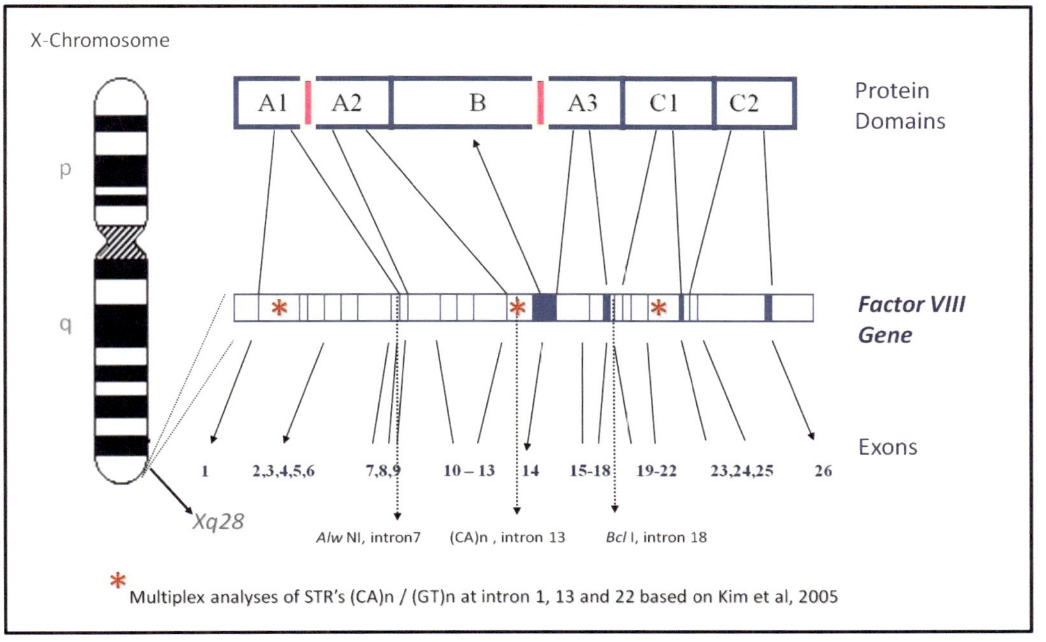

Fig. 3. Intragenic polymorphisms of *factor VIII* gene used for carrier diagnosis in hemophilia A in the Mexican population

In the case of hemophilia B we used four RFLPs of *factor IX* gene in order of heterozygosity: *Hha*I-3′ terminal region (50%); *Nru*I and *Sal*I in the promoter region (40-20%); *Taq*I-intron D (30%) and *Hinf*I-intron A (25%). Together the polymorphisms are highly informative and most families (>90%) are diagnosed for carrier status using these markers (Mantilla-Capacho et al., 2005).

4.3 Detection of common mutations in hemophilia A

The inversion of intron 22 in *factor VIII* gene is the most common mutation in hemophilia A. It is the cause of the severe form of the disease due to the inversion of *factor VIII* gene at intron 22 and its disruption from the rest of the gene caused by an intrachromosomal recombination of a region at intron 22 and two copies located at 400 kb toward the telomeric region (Lakich et al., 1993; Naylor et al., 1993). This rearrangement is responsible for 40-50% of severe hemophilia A cases. A similar mechanism at intron 1 accounts for 1-5% of severe cases (Bagnall et al., 2002).

Using the method of long-distance PCR (Liu et al., 1998) we found a frequency of 45% of the intron 22 inversion in patients with severe hemophilia A. We did not find the intron 1 inversion in the Mexican population with severe hemophilia A (n=65) (Mantilla-Capacho et al., 2007). Intron 22 inversion as the complex rearrangement causing the absence of FVIII protein has been identified as a moderate genetic risk factor for inhibitor development in patients with the severe form of the disease (Mantilla-Capacho et al., 2007).

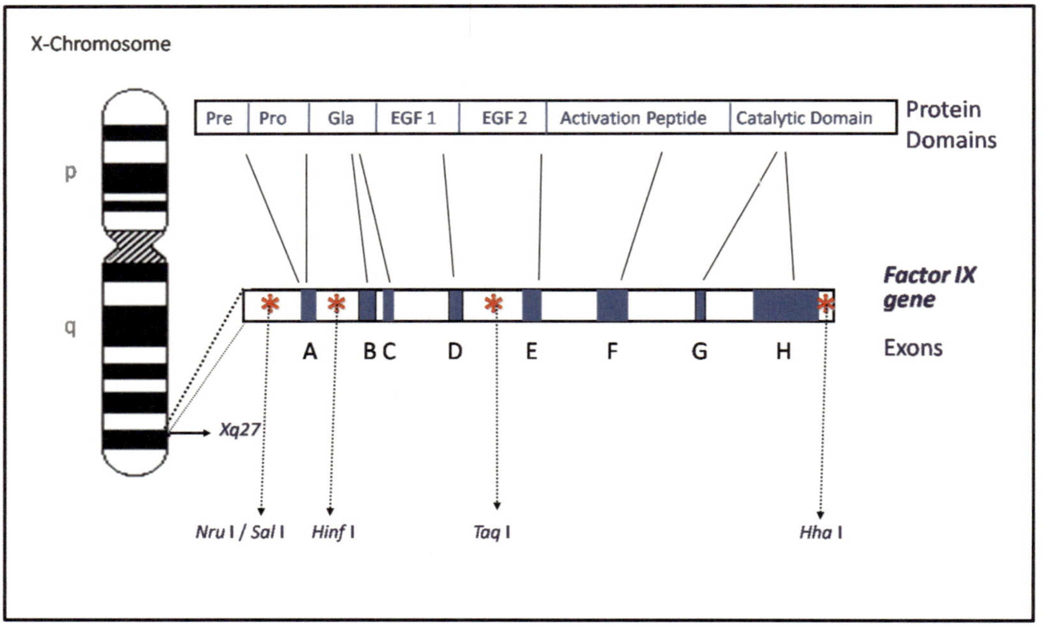

Fig. 4. Intragenic polymorphisms of *factor IX* gene used for carrier diagnosis in hemophilia B in the Mexican population

A new procedure was recently developed for the simultaneous detection of both inversions and the discrimination between distal and proximal rearrangements of intron 22 inversions (inv22-type 1 and inv22-type 2, respectively) by a novel inverse shifting PCR (IS-PCR) approach (Rossetti et al., 2008). This genotyping method includes the following: a) genomic digestion by *BclI* enzyme followed by b) self-ligation of the digested fragments containing the sequences of intron 22 of factor VIIII gene and their telomeric copies and c) a final PCR standard with different primers to detect normal and recombined fragments. The method also includes complementary diagnostic testing for detection of nondeleterious variants (normal products and duplications) produced by intron 22 rearrangements (Rossetti et al., 2008).

This procedure has recently been established in our laboratory and tested in a group of 24 patients with severe hemophilia A from independent families showing similar results in frequencies previously reported for the inversions in the Mexican population of severe hemophilia A patients (46% intron 22 inversion; 0% intron 1 inversion). From this study it was also possible to discriminate between both types of inv22. We found a frequency of 73% of type 1 inv22 and 27% of type 2 inv22 (Valdés-Galván, 2011). A high-quality DNA sample and the self-ligation step conditions are important in order to obtain consistent results. IS-PCR is the first-choice method for genetic analyses and carrier diagnosis in familial and sporadic cases of severe hemophilia A.

5. Hemorrhage phenotype attenuation in hemophilia by prothrombotic genes

In monogenic diseases such as hemophilia A and B, good correlation is expected between genotype and phenotype, i.e., type of mutation in *factor VIII* and *factor IX* genes causing

functional deficiency of the respective proteins to determine clinical severity. This is valid at the biochemical level (clotting activity) but not directly related to the bleeding symptoms in patients because there is clinical variability due to components other than deficient FVIII and FIX (White, 2001).

Different reports and meta-analyses have shown that, despite similar mutations in *factor VIII* or *factor IX* genes, there is an expected clinical variability in hemophilia. This is due to natural anticoagulant and fibrinolytic genes (Shetty et al., 2007, as cited in López-Jiménez et al., 2009) or the concomitant presence of mutations causative of prothrombotic risk factors (Factor V G1691A and Factor II 20210A). These cause the attenuation of hemorrhagic symptoms such as onset of bleeding episodes and frequency of hemarthroses as well as treatment requirements (Nichols et al., 1996; Kurnick et al., 2007; Tizzano et al., 2002; as cited in López-Jiménez et al., 2009) and from an extensive review of literature, FVLeiden has demonstrated to decrease hemophilia severity most consistently (Van Dijk et al., 2004). These studies have also demonstrated thrombosis risk in hemophilia patient carriers of prothrombotic genes such as reported for a patient with hemophilia B who suffered a venous thromboembolism as a result of exposure to high doses of replacement treatment during a surgical procedure (Pruthi et al., 2000).

Descriptive studies of hemophilia A and B families with some affected members with a striking attenuation of bleeding symptoms have demonstrated evidence of attenuation of bleeding phenotype attributable to the presence of prothombotic markers such as Factor V G1691A and Factor II 20210A. To some extent, these are also related to allelic polymorphisms of the methylenetetrahydrofolate-reductase (MTHFR) gene related to the activity of the enzyme (C677T) and the regulatory domain (A1298C). From a study in Mexican families with hemophilia A and B, the effect of Factor V G1691A and Factor II 20210A was demonstrated in the attenuation of hemorrhagic symptoms in hemophilia patients (López-Jiménez et al., 2009). The attenuation of hemophilia phenotype was mainly observed in the delay of bleeding symptom onset and secondly in a lower frequency of bleeding episodes (López-Jiménez et al., 2009). There was no evidence of an additional effect of attenuation on hemorrhagic symptoms by MTHFR polymorphisms, confirming the main contribution of Factor V G1691A and Factor II 20210A mutations, which are modulating genes of the hemophilia phenotype. On the basis of the feasible molecular analysis by routine PCR of prothrombotic genes and their relative frequency in different populations (1-5%), screening is recommended in those hemophilia patients with noncongruent clinical behavior in regard to severity by clotting activity of factor VIII or factor IX proteins.

6. Thrombin generation assay to evaluate clinical severity and treatment response in hemophilia

In search of objective criteria for the classification of clinical severity in hemophilia and prognostic factors with regard to treatment response in patients, functional approaches reflecting overall hemostatic behavior have shown important usefulness in providing parameters for clinical evaluation and investigation. The fundamental premise of the method is based on thrombin as a central molecule of coagulation whose increase or decrease reflects any alteration from the hemostasis equilibrium caused by hemorrhagic or thrombotic factors. The thrombin generation assay (TGA) was originally analyzed as a research source beginning in the 1950s with significant limitations due to labor-intensive requirements by subsampling and its application being restricted to only very specialized laboratories (Hemker, 2000).

Subsequently, Hemker and coworkers (2003) continued the research and improvement of the method until automation in calibrated automated thrombography.

6.1 TGA and correlation with clinical severity in hemophilia

Using calibrated automated thrombography, we studied 23 hemophilia A patients from nine families. Correlation analysis was done for clinical severity (according to an annual number of hemarthroses) and by the clotting activity of FVIII. The study showed that TGA was not able to discriminate differences among familial members but showed correlation with the general bleeding tendency of the clinical severity of patients according to FVIII:C levels (Beltrán-Miranda et al., 2005). Different parameters of the TGA may be useful to correlate with clinical severity in addition to endogenous thrombin potential (ETP), such as the peak and rate of thrombin generation.

6.2 TGA and inhibitor behavior in hemophilia A patients

In search of prognostic factors of treatment response in patients positive to inhibitors, we describe the kinetic study of FVIII:C inhibitors and TGA *in vitro* in poor platelet plasma (PPP) of hemophilia A patients positive to inhibitors to correlate with clinical parameters of response to available treatments in Mexico (Luna-Záizar, 2008).

The activity of FVIII:C in plasma was measured by one-stage clotting method and inhibitors to factor VIII was investigated using the Nijmegen-Bethesda method. Inhibitor kinetics was determined by plasma dilutions. TGA was measured in the inhibitor-positive PPP previously spiked and incubated with two treatments: FVIII and Activated Prothrombin Complex Concentrate (APCC, FEIBA™) by the Calibrated Automated Thrombography. Response to treatment by clinical criterion was assessed by 30 hematologists from 25 health institutions according to a questionnaire that assessed specific parameters of reduction of bleeding and improvement from the damage by decreasing pain and inflammation. We detected inhibitor antibodies in 71 patients (37.8%): 46 high responders (5-1,700 NB-U/mL) and 25 low-responders (0.6-4.7 NB-U/mL). When the plasmas of patients with high-responding inhibitors were incubated with the therapeutic product we found some changes in the thrombogram parameters. We found a significant association between inhibitor type and clinical treatment response to FVIII ($p=0.0003$, $n=42$) and between type kinetics vs. FVIII response evaluated with ETP ($p=0.0021$, $n=47$).

Concordance of FVIII response under clinical criteria and ETP was 71%, 86% and 67% among patients with type I, II and III inhibitors, respectively. The inhibitor kinetics was a prognostic parameter of response to FVIII replacement therapy in 74% of the patients. The change in the ETP parameter showed a relationship between inhibitor type and clinical treatment response. TGA permitted an individual evaluation of treatment response and showed usefulness such as objective criterion of responsiveness for a better selection of therapeutic resources, such as observed in one studied patient (Figure 5) (Luna-Záizar, 2008).

Other studies have also demonstrated the usefulness of TGA for monitoring treatment response to bypassing agents in patients positive to inhibitors in approaches carried out *in vivo* (Varadi et al, 2003 as cited in Dargaud et al., 2005) and *ex vivo* (Dargaud et al., 2005, 2010), which use the TGA as an important tool for direct clinical application in regard to medical decisions such as treatment doses and management of hemophilia patients with inhibitors.

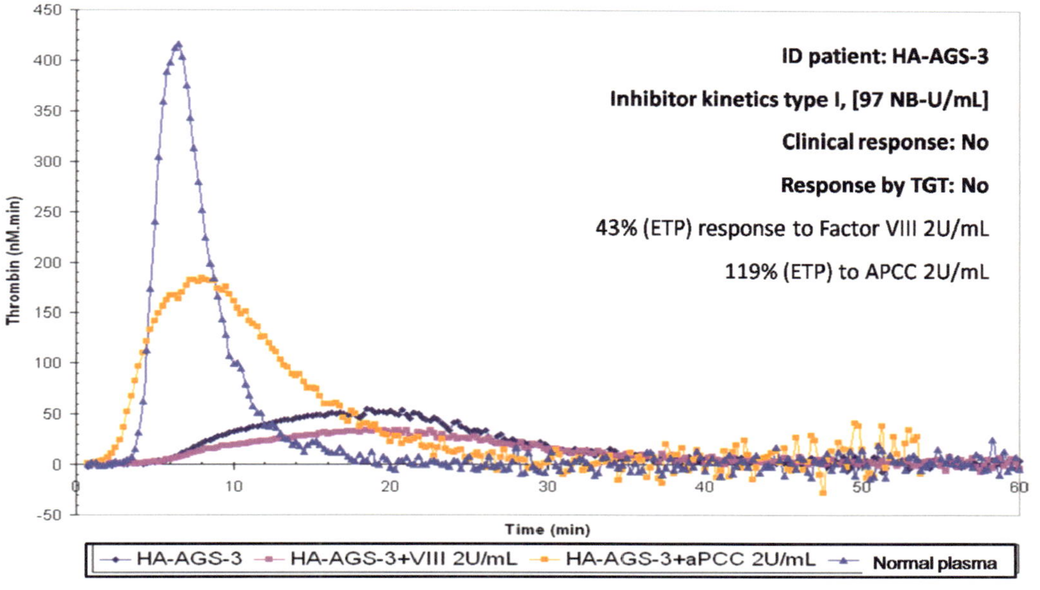

Fig. 5. TGA parameters in a hemophilia A patient positive to inhibitors and treatment response. Response to factor VIII and APCC by ETP increment from basal levels evaluated in platelet poor plasma of hemophilia A patients with inhibitors (Luna-Záizar, 2008).

7. X-chromosome inactivation pattern in hemophilia carriers with bleeding symptoms

Because hemophilia A and B are X-linked recessive disorders, males are affected, whereas females are carriers and usually asymptomatic due to the lyonization phenomenon. The lyonization process allows expression of only one allele of the genes located in the X active chromosome. For this reason, females are mosaic for the expression of maternal and paternal alleles and each chromosome contributes ~50% of gene expression (Puck & Willard, 1998), which is sufficient to prevent females from the manifestations of the disease. X-chromosome inactivation is a stochastic event that occurs early in female embryonic development to achieve dosage compensation with males. Certain genetic mechanisms affect the normal process causing a skewed X-inactivation pattern that has clinical relevance in female carriers of X-linked recessive disorders such as hemophilia (Mundo-Ayala & Jaloma-Cruz, 2008).

In probabilistic terms, the X-inactivation process follows a normal distribution pattern; however, it is possible to observe skewed and extremely skewed values (Amos-Landgraf et al., 2006). In some instances, skewness is due to the variation of the process itself when the inactivation ratio among X chromosomes is close to the mean value (75:25) or (80:20). Skewness higher than these proportions may indicate a genetic cause (Amos-Landgraf et al., 2006).

Genetic mechanisms that can explain extreme skewness of the X-inactivation process include mutations in genes that participate in the lyonization phenomenon. A mutation on

the promoter region of the XIST gene has been described that affects the randomness of the process resulting in a skewed X inactivation (Plenge et al., 1997; Tompkins et al., 2002).

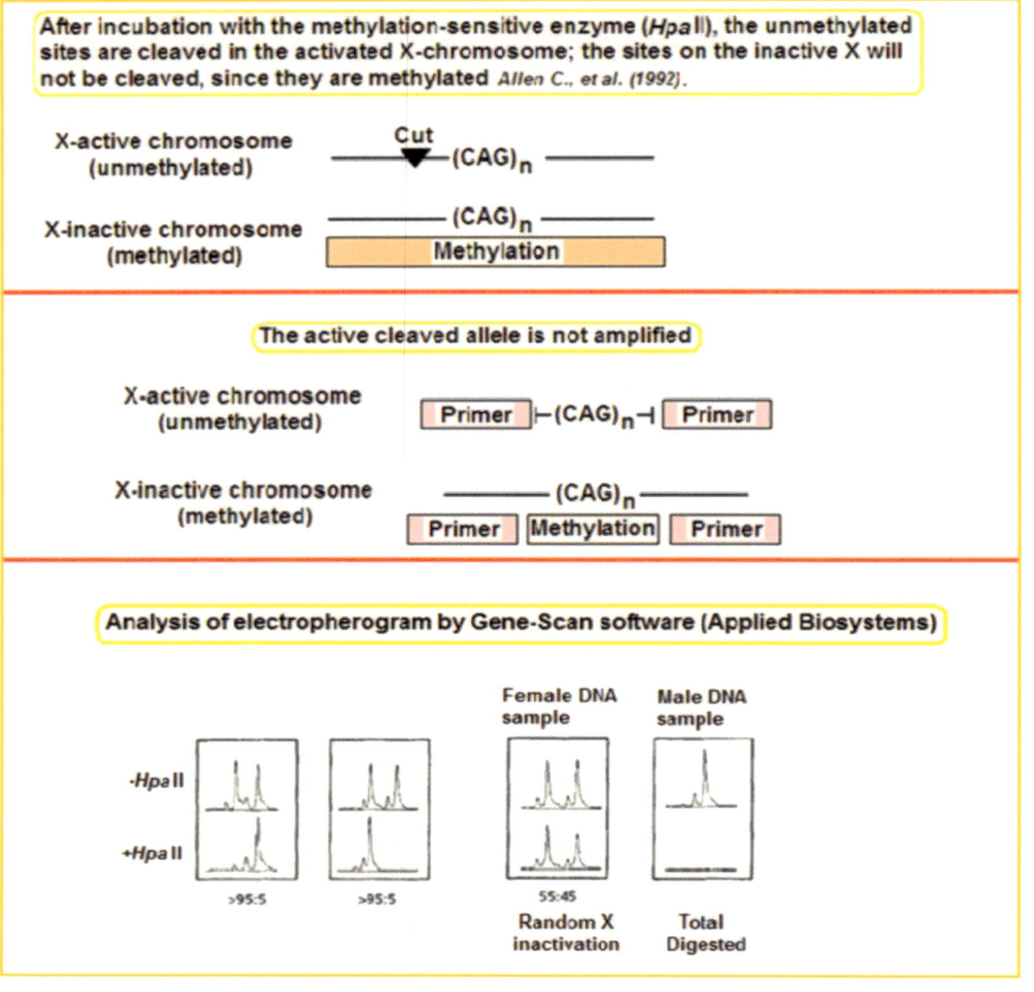

Fig. 6. Scheme of the HUMARA assay. Analysis of the X-inactivation pattern using DNA samples and the Gene-Scan software (Applied Biosystems®).

7.1 Molecular diagnosis of skew in the X-chromosome inactivation pattern in symptomatic hemophilia carriers

A symptomatic hemophilia carrier may request genetic counseling due to the presence of bleeding such as menorrhagia, epistaxis, bruising, gingivitis, etc. (Mundo-Ayala & Jaloma-Cruz, 2008). In case of symptoms in a hemophilia B carrier and after ruling out von Willebrand disease (in a symptomatic carrier of hemophilia A) or chromosomal anomalies such as Turner syndrome to explain the bleeding symptoms, geneticists and molecular biologists should consider analysis of the X-inactivation pattern in the DNA samples of the patient and her parents (Mundo-Ayala & Jaloma-Cruz, 2008).

The gold standard for the analysis of the X-inactivation pattern is the human androgen receptor assay (HUMARA) developed by Allen et al. (1992). We recently used a modified protocol for automatic genotyping of HUMARA by fluorescent Genescan® described by Karasawa et al. (2001) with some modifications to achieve a precise reading in the GC-rich region of the polymorphic region of HUMARA (Ishiyama et al., 2003) and to improve the yield of PCR product and digestion to discriminate the active/inactive alleles by methylation (Mundo-Ayala & Jaloma-Cruz, 2008; Mundo-Ayala, 2010). The methodology is illustrated in Figure 6 and our group has described it in detail for the automatic fluorescent Genescan® (Mundo-Ayala & Jaloma-Cruz, 2008; Mundo-Ayala, 2010). Use of this technique in bleeding carriers and females with hemophilia allows identifying whether their hemorrhagic symptoms are due to an unfavorable lyonization.

7.2 Analysis of a Mexican hemophilia A family with a symptomatic carrier

We describe the study of X-chromosome inactivation pattern in a family with hemophilia A and a symptomatic carrier (Figure 7). Members of this family are affected males, and two of four sisters (II:6 and II:7) were confirmed as carriers after molecular diagnosis by *factor VIII* polymorphisms. Sister (II:7) is a symptomatic carrier who presented clinical manifestations of hemophilia A and a significantly reduced level of FVIII:C (2.5%). Using molecular analysis to determine the X-inactivation pattern, a nonrandom X inactivation was found. The results showed that the healthy X chromosome inherited from the father was preferentially inactive, whereas the affected chromosome from maternal origin was expressed in ~96% of the patient's total organism (Mundo-Ayala, 2010).

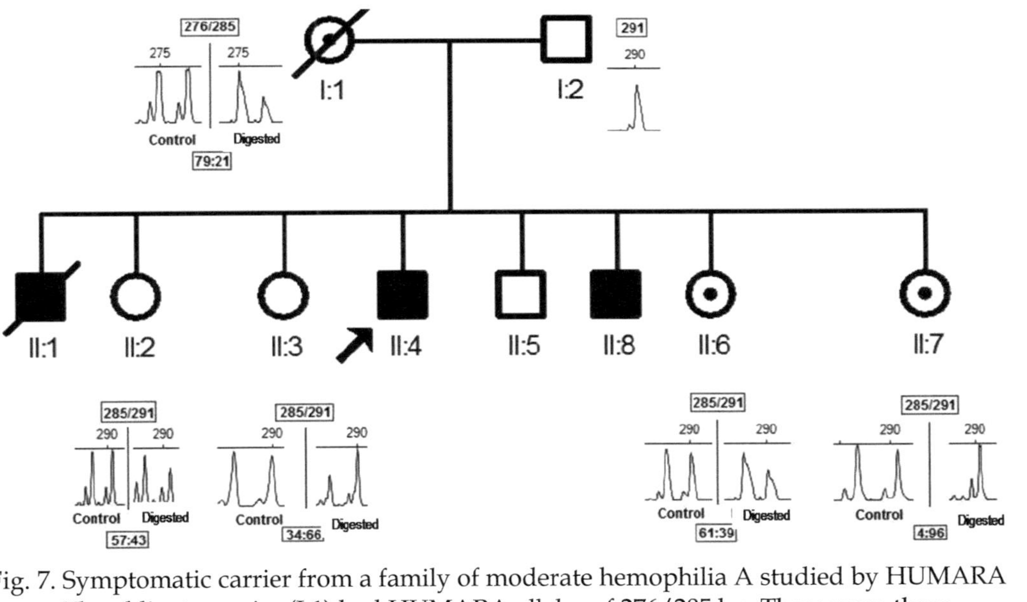

Fig. 7. Symptomatic carrier from a family of moderate hemophilia A studied by HUMARA assay. The obligate carrier (I:1) had HUMARA alleles of 276/285 bp. There were three affected males; the propositus (II:4) is indicated with an arrow. There were four females; two (II:6, II:7) were carriers of hemophilia A as confirmed by molecular diagnosis. Symptomatic carrier (II:7) showing an extreme X-inactivation pattern that explains her bleeding manifestations due to the preferential inactivation of the paternal X chromosome.

Clinical bleeding manifestations in the symptomatic carrier (II:7) of this family with hemophilia A occur as a result of the nonrandom X inactivation pattern, which favorably silences the healthy X chromosome inherited from her father. After a negative result of mutations at the promoter region of XIST gene, the molecular origin remains unknown of the skewness in the symptomatic carrier (Mundo-Ayala, 2010).

From the study of different symptomatic carriers of hemophilia from Mexican families, we conclude that it is important to provide genetic counseling due to the possibility of inheriting a nonrandom pattern of X-chromosome inactivation.

Clinical implications from the skewed pattern of X-chromosome must be considered for genetic counseling and hematological control in symptomatic carriers. Furthermore, analysis of X-inactivation pattern is necessary for understanding the human X-chromosome inactivation process (Mundo-Ayala & Jaloma-Cruz, 2008).

8. Conclusions

The various studies presented in this chapter emphasize the importance of a comprehensive overview in hemophilia, considering multiple interactions among genes, metabolic pathways and different approaches including molecular data, biochemical analysis and clinical aspects. All these factors are important in order to consider an integrative evaluation of the clinical aspects of hemophilia so as to improve medical management and to obtain prognostic factors for clinical behavior and treatment response.

9. Acknowledgements

The authors of this chapter dedicate all the work described here carried out during 17 years to the **Federación de Hemofilia de la República Mexicana, A.C**. and to all the affiliated associations in the country, especially to the Jalisco Association **"Unidad y Desarrollo, Hermanos con Hemofilia, A.C."**, with hope that all the developed research may contribute to the welfare and improvement in the quality of life of Mexican hemophilia patients and their families.

Our deepest gratitude to **Dr. María Amparo Esparza Flores**, to **Dr. Janet Margarita Soto Padilla**, hematologists-pediatricians, and to all Mexican hematologists for their invaluable work for the health of hemophilia patients and to all those who have contributed to our research.

10. References

Amos-Landgraf, J.M., Cottle, A., Plenge, R.M., Friez M., Schwartz, C.E., Longshore, J., & Willard, H.F. (2006). X Chromosome-inactivation patterns of 1,005 phenotypically unaffected females. *The American Journal of Human Genetics*. Vol. 79. No. 3. (September 2006). pp. 493-499.

Bagnall, R.D., Waseem, N., Green, P.M., & Giannelli, F. (2002). Recurrent inversion breaking intron 1 of the factor VIII gene is a frequent cause of severe hemophilia A. *Blood*. Vol. 99. pp. 168-174.

Barrowcliffe, T.W. (2004). Monitoring haemophilia severity and treatment: new or old laboratory tests? (2004). *Haemophilia*. Vol. 10. No. (Suppl. 4). pp. 109-114.

Beltrán-Miranda, C.P., Khan, A., Jaloma-Cruz, A.R., & Laffan, M. (2005). Thrombin generation and genotype-phenotype correlation in haemophilia A. *Haemophilia.* Vol. 11. (March 2005). pp. 326-334.

Bowen, DJ. (2002). Review. Haemophilia A and haemophilia B: molecular insights. *Journal of Clinical Pathology: Molecular Pathology.* Vol. 55 (May 2001), pp. 1–18.

Dargaud, Y., Lienhart, A., Meunier, S., Hequet, O., Chavanne, H.,Chamouard, V., Marin, S., & Negrier, C. (2005). Major surgery in a severe haemophilia A patient with high titre inhibitor: use of the thrombin generation test in the therapeutic decision. Case Report. *Haemophilia.* Vol. 11. (July 2005). pp. 552–558.

Dargaud, Y., Lienhart, A. & Negrier, C. (2010). Prospective assessment of thrombin generation test for dose monitoring of bypassing therapy in hemophilia patients with inhibitors undergoing elective surgery. *Blood.* Vol. 116. No. 25. (September 2010). Pp. 5734-5737.

Enjolras, N., Plantier, J-L., Rodriguez, M-H., Rea, M., Attali, O., Vinciguerra, C., & Negrier C. (2004). Two novel mutations in EGF-like domains of human factor IX dramatically impair intracellular processing and secretion. *Journal of Thrombosis and Haemostasis.* Vol. 2. No. 7 (July 2004). pp. 1143-1154.

González Ramos, I.A., Mundo-Ayala, J.N., & Jaloma-Cruz, A.R. (2010). Carrier diagnosis of hemophilia a by fluorescent multiplex PCR. (05P10). Vol. 16. No. Suppl. 4. p. 17. Carriers and prenatal Issues. *Hemophilia.* XXIX International Congress of the World Federation of Hemophilia. Buenos Aires, Argentina, July 2010.

Hemker, H.C., Giesen, P.L., Ramjee, M., Wagenvoord, R., & Béguin, S. (2000). The thrombogram: monitoring thrombin generation in platelet rich plasma. *Thrombosis and Haemostasis.* Vol. 83. No. 4. pp. 589-591.

Hemker, H.C., Giesen, P., Al Dieri, R., Regnault, V., De Smedt, E., Wagenvoord, R., Lecompte, T., & Bèguin, S. (2003). Calibrated automated thrombin generation measurement in clotting plasma. *Pathophysiol Haemost Thromb.* Vol. 33. pp. 4-15.

Ishiyama, K., Chuhjo, T., Wang, H., Yachie A., Omine, M., & Nakao, S. (2003). Polyclonal hematopoiesis maintained in patients with bone marrow failure harboring a minor population of paroxysmal nocturnal hemoglobinuria-type cells. *Blood.* Vol. 102. No. 4. (August 2003). pp. 1211-1216.

Jaloma-Cruz, A.R., Scaringe, W.A., Drost, J.B., Roberts, S., Li, X., Barros-Núñez, P., Figuera, L.E., Rivas, F., Cantú J.M., & Sommer S.S. (2000). Nine independent F9 mutations in the Mexican hemophilia B population: nonrandom recurrences of point mutation events in the human germline. *Human Mutation, Mutation in Brief.* Vol. 15 (Dec 1999), pp. 116-117.

Kim, J-W., Park, S-Y., Kim, Y-M., Kim, J-M., Kim, D-J., & Ryu H-M. (2005). Identification of new dinucleotide-repeat polymorphisms in factor VIII gene using fluorescent PCR. *Haemophilia.* Vol. 11 (December 2004), pp. 38-42.

Koeberl, D.D., Bottema, C.D.K., Ketterling R.P., Bridge, P.J., Lillicrapt D.P., & Sommer S.S. (1990). Mutations causing hemophilia B: direct estimate of the underlying rates of spontaneous germ-line transitions, deletions, and transversions in a human gene. *American Journal of Human Genetics.* Vol. 47 (March 1990), pp. 202-217. ISSN 0002-9297/90/4702-0005.

Lakich, D., Kazazian, H.H., Antonarakis, S.E., & Gitschier, J. (1993). Inversions disrupting the factor VIII gene are common cause of severe Haemophilia A. *Nature Genetics.* Vol. 5, pp. 236-241.

Leuer, M., Oldenburg, J., Lavergne, J-M, Ludwig, M., Fregin, M., Eigel, A., Ljung, R., Goodeve, A., Peake, I., & Olek K. (2001). Somatic mosaicism in hemophilia A: a fairly common event. *American Journal of Human Genetics.* Vol. 69 (July 2001), pp. 75–87. ISSN 0002-9297/2001/6901-0009.

Liu, Q., Nozari, G., & Sommer, S.S. (1998). Single-tube polymerase chain reaction for rapid diagnosis of the inversion hotspot of mutation in haemophilia A. *Blood.* Vol. 92. pp. 1458-1459.

López-Jimenez, J.J., Beltrán-Miranda, C.P., Mantilla-Capacho, J.M., Esparza-Flores, M.A., López-González, L.C., & Jaloma-Cruz A.R. (2009). Clinical variability of haemophilia A and B in Mexican families by factor V Leiden G1691A, prothrombin G20210A and MTHFR C677T/A1298C. *Haemophilia.* Vol. 15. pp. 1342-1345.

Luna-Záizar, H. (2008). Cinética de inactivación al factor VIII y generación de trombina como pronóstico de respuesta al tratamiento y asociación de marcadores genéticos con el desarrollo de inhibidores en pacientes con hemofilia a grave. *Ph.D thesis on Human Genetics.* Centro Universitario de Ciencias de la Salud, Universidad de Guadalajara. Guadalajara, Jalisco, México.

Mantilla-Capacho, J.M., Beltrán-Miranda, C.P., & Jaloma-Cruz, A.R. (2005). Diagnóstico molecular en pacientes y portadoras de hemofilia A y B. *Gaceta Médica de México.* Vol. 141, No. 1, pp. 69-71.

Mantilla-Capacho, J.M., Beltrán-Miranda, C.P., Luna-Záizar H., Aguilar-López, L.B., Esparza-Flores, M.A., López-Guido, B., Troyo-Sanromán R., & Jaloma-Cruz, A.R. (2007). Frequency of intron 1 and 22 inversions of *factor VIII* gene in Mexican patients with severe hemophilia A. *American Journal of Hematology.* Vol. 82 (January 2007). pp. 283-287.

Mantilla-Capacho, J.M., Enjolras, N., Négrier, C., & Jaloma-Cruz, A.R. (2008). Intracellular trafficking analysis of C111Y and C111S mutations of factor IX identified in Mexican patients with severe hemophilia B. *Hemophilia.* Vol. 14. No. Suppl. 2. p. 65. Molecular Genetics of Bleeding Disorders. (11 FP 05). XXVIII International Congress of the World Federation of Hemophilia. Istanbul, Turkey June 1-5, 2008.

Mundo-Ayala, J.N., & Jaloma-Cruz, A.R. (2008). Evaluación del patrón de inactivación del cromosoma X en portadoras sintomáticas y mujeres con hemofilia. *Gaceta Médica de México.* Vol. 144. pp. 171-174.

Mundo-Ayala, J.N. (2010). Patrón de inactivación del cromosoma X y mutaciones en el promotor del gen *XIST* en portadoras sintomáticas de hemofilia A y B. *Ph.D. thesis on Human Genetics.* Centro Universitario de Ciencias de la Salud. Universidad de Guadalajara. Guadalajara, Jalisco, 2010.

Naylor J., Brinke, A., Hassock, S., Green, P.M., & Giannelli, F. (1993). Characteristic mRNA abnormality found in half the patients with severe haemophilia A is due to large inversions. *Human Molecular Genetics.* Vol. 2, pp. 1773-1778.

Plenge, R.M., Hendrich, B.D., Schwartz, C., Arena, J.F., Naumova, A., Sapienza, C., Winter R.M. and Willard, H.F. (1997). A promoter mutation in the *XIST* gene in two unrelated families with skewed X-chromosome inactivation. *Nat Genet.* Vol. 17. pp. 353-356.

Pruthi, R.K., Heit, J.A., Green, M.M., Emiliusen, L.M., Nichols, W.L., Wilke, J.L., Gastineau, D.A. (2000). Venous thromboembolism after hip fracture surgery in a patient with hemophilia B and factor V Arg 506 Gln (factor V Leiden). *Haemophilia*. Vol. 6. (April 2000). pp. 631–634.

Puck, J.M., & Willard, H.F. (1998). X Inactivation in females with X-linked disease. *The New England Journal of Medicine*. Vol. 338, (January 1998). pp. 325-328.

Rossetti, L.C., Radic, C.P., Larripa, I.B., & De Brasi, C.D. (2008). Developing a new generation of tests for genotyping hemophilia-causative rearrangements involving *int22h* and *int1h* hotspots in the factor VIII gene. *Journal of Thrombosis and Haemostasis*. Vol. 6. (January 2008). pp. 830-836.

Sommer, S.S. (1995). Recent human germ-line mutation: inferences from patients with hemophilia B. *Trends in Genetics*. Vol. 11, No. 4. (April 1995). pp. 141-147.

Tomkins, D.J., McDonald, H.L., Farrel, S.A., Brown, C.J. (2002). Lack of expression of *XIST* from a small ring X chromosome containing the *XIST* locus in a girl with short stature, facial dysmorphism and developmental delay. *European Journal of Human Genetics*. Vol. 10. (November 2001). pp. 44-51.

Valdés-Galván, M.J. (2011). Detección de las inversiones de los intrones 1 y 22 por PCR inversa cambiante (*IS-PCR*) en pacientes con hemofilia A grave. *Masters degree thesis in Clinic Biomedicine*. Escuela de Ciencias, Departamento de Ciencias Químico-Biológicas. Universidad de las Américas Puebla. San Andrés Cholula, Puebla, México.

Van Dijk, K., Van der Bom, J.G., Fischer, K. Grobbee D.E., Van der Berg, H.M. (2004). Do prothrombotic factors influence clinical phenotype of severe haemophilia? A review of the literature. *Thrombosis and Haemostasis*. Vol. 92. (June 2004). pp. 305–310.

White, G.C. II, Rosendaal, F., Aledort, L.M., Lusher, J.M., Rothschild, C., & Ingerslev, J., on behalf of the Factor VIII and Factor IX Subcommittee. (2001). Definitions in hemophilia: Recommendation of the Scientific Subcommittee on Factor VIII and Factor IX of the Scientific and Standardization Committee of the International Society on Thrombosis and Haemostasis. *Thrombosis and Haemostasis*. Vol. 85, p. 560.

3

From Genotype to Phenotype – When the Parents Ask the Question

Rumena Petkova[1], Stoian Chakarov[2] and Varban Ganev[2]
[1]*Scientific Technological Service Ltd.*
[2]*Sofia University "St. Kliment Ohridski"*
Bulgaria

1. Introduction

Bleeding disorders often present with different degrees of severity, ranging from very mild to very severe. Clinical presentation is not always correlated with the grade of the molecular defect and the disruption it causes to the gene/s in question. This is especially true for circulating coagulation factor deficiencies where even 1-2 % difference between levels of the deficient factor may result in significant variations in the clinical presentation. It is often the case that the residual level of factor does not serve as a reliable predictor of the clinical course in the particular patient. This is related to a number of reasons, including timing and accuracy of level measurement, antigenic properties/activity ratio of the deficient factor, nature of the molecular defect, presence of factors augmenting or alleviating the bleeding tendency (such as antibodies to the deficient factor, co-inherited prothrombotic risk factors, etc.). Therefore, prognostication of disease course in young children and for the possibility of recurrence of the bleeding phenotype in the family could present quite a challenge to the genetic counselor. Nevertheless, this aspect of disease coping is very important to the family undergoing genetic counseling for haemophilia as it might influence their motivation for seeking adequate therapy and trying novel treatments, might induce overprotectiveness towards the affected child and most definitely could modify the family's future reproductive plans (having one ill child and a grim perspective for the disease course usually does not encourage having more children). The ability to answer the questions of the parents about the prospective course of the disease with an acceptable degree of reliability is a crucial component of genetic counseling for haemophilia and requires gathering and processing a lot of information in order to produce a reliable image of what could be expected and what could be avoided.

2. Factors that contribute to the haemophilic phenotype

The avalanche stopping in its tracks a few feet above the cowering village behaves not only unnaturally but unethically.
Vladimir Nabokov, Pnin (1957)

Haemophilia A is a common (affecting 1:8000-1:10000 males) bleeding disorder caused by a deficiency of Factor VIII, a cofactor for the activated blood clotting factor IXa (Kazazian et al., 1995). The latter is a serine protease, activating factor X in the coagulation cascade, which

ultimately leads to the conversion of prothrombin to thrombin and to formation of a fibrin clot. Deficiency of Factor IX produces haemophilia B, a more rarely encountered (approximately 1:40000 males) bleeding disorder which is practically identical to haemophilia A in terms of clinical presentation as both factors act in the same biochemical pathway.

It could be expected that the level of residual factor would be inversely proportional to the grade of clinical severity, i.e. the lower the level of residual factor, the more severe the bleeding tendency. The level of the deficient factor is calculated as a ratio of the coagulation capability of the patient's plasma compared to a plasma pool of healthy males (taken as a 100 % reference point). Generally, haemophilia in patients with levels of 0-1 % of the deficient factor is classified as severe, 2-5 % as moderate and 6-40 % as mild. Patients with undetectably low levels of the deficient factor or up to 1 % are at risk of bleeding after minor injury or even without apparent precipitating event (also called spontaneous bleeding).

Bleeding tendency in severe haemophilia is usually noted early in life (around the age when the baby starts walking) or even in the immediate neonatal period because of cephalhaematoma after assisted delivery by means of forceps or vacuum extraction. Patients with levels within the 2-5 % range exhibit a heterogeneous spectrum of bleeding severity, ranging from indistinguishable from severe cases to mild, which becomes apparent only after serious challenge (e.g. dental manipulations). Patients in the mild category (6 % and upwards) are usually identified as haemophiliacs later in life (up to the fourth and fifth decade) and will usually bleed profusely only following a significant precipitating event (e.g. surgery, serious injury, etc.).

Severe haemophilia accounts for about 50 % of all the cases that come to clinical attention, moderate cases are about 40 % and, respectively, mild haemophilia makes up for the remaining 10 %. It is believed that severe cases are overrepresented in the statistics at the expense of milder forms as patients with severe bleeding tendency are more likely to be entered into the relevant registries.

It is more often than not that the patient presents with signs and symptoms of bleeding tendency of certain grade and subsequent clotting factor level measurements do not support the clinical findings. There are a number of reasons that might explain the discrepancy and each and every one of these must be checked and verified before a reliable assessment of disease severity and prognostication of the course of the disease could be made.

2.1 Errors in determining the level of residual factor

The first and foremost of the sources of errors in determination of clinical severity is inadequate timing of the coagulation factor level measurement. Often, families are motivated to visit the genetic counseling unit because of newly discovered pregnancy or because they are planning a pregnancy. It is often the case that the family does not actually know whether it is haemophilia A or haemophilia B that presents in their family and any laboratory data of a correctly taken blood sample from the index patient might not be immediately available. Thus, a sample taken from a haemophilic male 'at random' might produce spurious results. As a rule, errors of this type are biased towards measuring higher level of the deficient coagulation factor because of recent transfusion of plasma or blood clotting factor preparations. In our practice we had one haemophilic boy who repeatedly measured over 10 % of factor VIII when blood was taken for genetic analysis and some of it was tested for Factor VIII activity by two-stage assay. Since the patient had several spontaneous bleeding incidents on record, further investigation of the boy's medical history was carried out. As it turned out, the boy liked competitive sports and his family regularly

requested a transfusion of factor VIII preparations at their local haemophilia center but chose not to share this information with the genetic counselor. Had the case not been thoroughly investigated, genetic analysis for most common defects causing severe haemophilia A would not have been chosen as first option in genetic analysis and the causative mutation would not have been discovered in time.

There is also the question of whether the circulating residual clotting factor has adequate biochemical activity in vivo or not. Back in 1968, the antigenic properties of the deficient factor were also included as a component in the laboratory testing panel for haemophilia A and B (Roberts et al., 1968; Zimmermann & Edgington, 1973), broadening the classification of haemophilia forms to CRM (cross-reacting material) positive or CRM - negative. Later, Denson (1973) introduced the concept of FVIII:C (the biochemical activity of residual Factor VIII) versus FVIII:Ag (the antigenic properties of residual Factor VIII). Basically, it is the concept of presence of Factor VIII as an immunochemically recognizable protein but not as a cofactor activity. This might be the case when the underlying genetic defect in the Factor VIII gene produces a truncated or incorrectly folded protein. The majority of patients with severe haemophilia A have no detectable level of factor VIII protein in plasma (CRM-negative) but there are about 5 % of all severe patients that are CRM-positive (though the amount of CRM is usually reduced). Therefore, the assessment of the residual factor VIII activity (FVIII: C) ought to be always coupled with measurement of the FVIII:Ag so as to avoid biased results because of detection of the FVIII protein in the plasma. It is very important that clear instructions are given about what measures should be taken to avoid errors in measurement of coagulation factor levels, as an incorrect result might cause delays in genetic analysis. The latter could be irreparable in cases when a high-risk pregnancy is involved.

2.2 Antibodies to factor VIII

About 10-50 % of patients with haemophilia who have been treated with plasma transfusions and/or preparations of Factor VIII or IX ultimately develop antibodies (also called inhibitors) to the deficient clotting factor (de Biasi et al., 1994; Oldenburg et al., 2000; Ghosh & Shetty, 2009). This results in decreased therapeutic efficiency (with potentially fatal consequences for the patient if a major bleeding could not be managed properly) and increases the costs of treatment (as more units of the clotting factor are required to achieve the desired effect). It is generally believed that recombinant Factor VIII is more immunogenic that Factor VIII derived from pooled plasma (Aledort, 2004; Goudemand et al., 2006), but the results of a large cohort study carried out in 2007 (Gouw et al.) did not show an association between type of Factor VIII preparation and rate of development of antibodies to the clotting factor.

Generally it is the patients with severe haemophilia that develop inhibitors to Factor VIII followed by patients with moderate disease (Schwaab et al., 1995; d'Oiron et al., 2008). This is only logical as the types of mutations which cause severe disease are more likely to produce CRM-negative haemophilia (hence, the exogenous Factor VIII protein is viewed as 'foreign' by the immune system) or CRM-positive haemophilia with misfolded protein exposing unusual immunogenic epitopes (Oldenburg et al., 2002; Goodeve & Peake, 2003; Ragni et al., 2009).

It is hard to predict whether the particular patient will develop antibodies to the deficient coagulation factor. The inhibitor phenotype is usually constituted via a fine interplay of genetic and non-genetic factors, though it is dependent on the type of the causative

mutation (Tuddenham & Oldenburg, 1995; Astermark, 2010). Generally, it is safe to advise parents of a patient with mild haemophilia that development of antibodies would be unlikely. This, however, would not be the parent's prime concern anyway, as their child most probably would not need regular transfusions of Factor VIII-containing preparations. In a case of severe or moderate haemophilia it is not acceptable to recite bluntly the risk percentages of antibody formation to the family as most often this will not register as a chance to have an uncomplicated therapy course but, rather, as a risk to develop an untreatable condition. It is more advisable to gently induce the parents to record the number of units transfused each time and the number of times when an unexpected bleeding has called for a transfusion out of schedule. This way a reliable estimate could be obtained of whether the same amount of units per kg body weight results in the same correction of the coagulation defect over time.

In our practice we have observed only patients with severe disease develop anti-Factor VIII antibodies. In one case the genetic background was particularly interesting as there were two maternal first cousins with severe haemophilia A, one of which had very severe disease complicated by antibodies resulting in haemophilic arthropathy of both knee and ankle joints at the age of 11, while his cousin, aged 13, who apparently shared the same Factor VIII-gene disrupting mutation, only used Factor VIII-containing preparations at 'on demand' basis, typically less often than once in two months and had no major joint injury. At the time it was only possible to rule out Factor VIII inversions with breakpoints within the repeated intron 22 unit so the nature of the mutation remained unknown. Since the patients were first cousins and came from an ethnic group with a long-standing tradition of consanguineous marriages, there was a high chance that the two patients also shared common polymorphisms in other genes that play a role in the risk of inhibitor development. It is possible that the one cousin developed antibodies to Factor VIII because of more frequent encounters with this protein than the other cousin but the reason why one had more severe phenotype than the other was not identified.

In cases when one haemophilic child with antibodies to the deficient clotting factor is already born, families are typically very reluctant to opt for another child as the presence of inhibitors seem to compromise the only possible therapy option. It is up to the genetic counselor to explain the risks of another case of antibody-complicated haemophilia to the family and to order additional tests if needed, such as HLA typing and/or IL-10 and TNF-alpha polymorphism typing (Hay et al., 1997; Pavlova et al., 2009; Chaves at al., 2010). In one of our cases, there was a 21 g. w. pregnancy with a male foetus in a woman who has had already one son with severe haemophilia A complicated by high-titer antibodies to Factor VIII. DNA from the index patient was unavailable, so the nature of the mutation causing haemophilia in the family was impossible to identify. The most common mutations causing haemophilia A (inversions with a breakpoint in intron 22) were not identified either in peripheral blood of the mother (so that germinative mosaicism could not be ruled out) or in the foetus. In the process of genetic counseling it became clear that the family was accepting of the fact that they might have another boy with haemophilia but the issue that worried them the most was the risk of developing inhibitors in the course of treatment. Since the index patient and the foetus from the present pregnancy had different biological fathers, the risk that they shared the same set of genes was less that the 25 % expected by pure chance in full siblings, therefore the risk that they had inherited the same HLA class II type that could contribute to the risk of inhibitor development was less that the norm for siblings. The mother did not carry the TNF-alpha G308A polymorphism. Therefore, since the causative mutation

could not be determined (at least not in the very condensed timeframe imposed upon us by the advanced pregnancy) the family was presented with the options of carrying the pregnancy to term and risking having another child with haemophila A (about 30 % risk based on the premise that about 30 % of first cases of haemophilia A are born to noncarrier women) that might eventually develop inhibitors to Factor VIII, or, or selectively terminating the pregnancy and risking abortion of a healthy male foetus (70 %). After weighing the risks the family opted for carrying pregnancy to term and actually had a healthy boy.

The incidence of antibody development in Bulgarian patients seems to be lower than usual (less than 10 %). We presume that this may be related to the practice of 'on-demand' treatment which was prevalent in Bulgaria until several years ago. With coagulation factor preparations getting more available to the patients, it could only be expected that the proportion of patients developing inhibitors to Factor VIII and Factor IX will reach the level reported elsewhere.

2.3 Nature of the causative mutation

A reasonable prediction of haemophilia phenotype and the course of the disease could be made based on the characteristics of the molecular defect. One must bear in mind, however, that the phenotype of the particular patient is not a direct function of the type of mutation but that additional genetic, epigenetic and environmental factors may play a role.

The gene for Factor VIII is situated in the distal part of the long arm of the X chromosome, Xq28 (Gitschier et al., 1984). The gene spans 186 Mb genomic DNA and comprises 26 exons ranging from 64 to 3106 bp in length. The resulting Factor VIII protein has a complicated domain structure with numerous sites for interaction with other molecules. Therefore, almost every hit within the coding regions of the gene and sometimes in the noncoding sequences may result in haemophilia phenotype. Up to the present moment over 1000 different mutations in factor VIII gene have been reported (Schwaab et al., 1991; Tuddenham et al., 1994, The Haemophila A Mutation Database, available from: http://hadb.org.uk/WebPages/PublicFiles/MutationSummary.htm, retrieved 14 May 2011). The mutation spectrum is heterogeneous with over 95 % of all mutations apart from the large gene rearrangements being single-nucleotide substitutions.

As a rule, nonsense mutations result in severe, CRM-negative haemophilia. Missense mutations may produce a variable phenotype, depending on the site where the mutation has occurred. Generally, mutations in the sequence coding for the A2 domain of the Factor VIII gene result in CRM - positive haemophilia with varying severity (Wakabayashi & Fay, 2008) as the A2 domain is responsible for the stability of the protein. Deletions of exons usually produces severe CRM-negative haemophilia A because of reading frame disruption except for deletion of exon 22 which results in an in-frame loss of 156 bp coding sequence (Youssouffian et al., 1987). and moderate haemophilia A. Deletions in the factor VIII gene are reported to be associated with increased tendency for inhibitor development because of incorrect protein folding resulting in exposure of immunogenic epitopes that are usually buried within the protein core (Youssouffian et al., 1987; Gouw et al., 2007, 2011). Specific mutation hotspots are 5-methylated cytosine residues which are readily deaminated to thymine (Youssoffian, 1986). These mutations usually result in introduction of premature stop codon (transition CGA→TGA) and, ultimately, in a truncated protein. The severity may vary depending on the site where the transition occurred but usually results in severe haemophilia with or without cross-reacting material as the truncated protein might be unstable in plasma (Reiner & Thompson, 1992).

2.3.1 Inversions with breakpoints in the 9.5 Kb repeated sequence in intron 22 of the factor VIII gene

About 50 % of haemophilia A cases are severe. In about half of these 50 % (25 % of all cases) the causative mutation does not affect the coding sequences of the gene but, rather, rearranges the gene in a way that precludes normal splicing across the exon 22 - exon 23 boundary of the gene (Naylor et al., 1992). Namely, this is a large inversion of the genomic portion containing exons 1-22 together as a unit which ultimately places them at considerable distance from exons 23-26. This is a randomly occurring event resulting from homologous recombination between inverted repeats located within the Factor VIII gene (intron 22) and outside the gene (Levinson et al., 1990, 1992).

Intron 22 of the Factor VIII gene is remarkable in more than one aspect. It is a very large intron (32.4 Kb) and possesses a CpG island of its own. The latter serves as an origin of transcription for two transcripts internal to the Factor VIII gene, termed F8A and F8B, and orientated, respectively, one opposite (F8A) and one parallel (F8B) to the direction of transcription of Factor VIII (Levinson et al., 1990, 1992). The sequence coding for F8A is located within a 9.5 Kb fragment which constitutes the repeated unit. There may be three or, rarely, four or more repeated units per X chromosome, one of which is always located inside intron 22 of the factor VIII gene and the others are extragenic, at distances of approximately 300 and 400 Kb from the Factor VIII gene. The repeated units have a very high degree of homology (over 99.9 %). During meiosis, it is likely that homologous sequences may mispair with their homologues on the same chromosome and serve as breakpoints for recombination. As the repeats outside Factor VIII gene are orientated in the opposite direction to the intragenic copy, the resulting rearrangement is an inversion of the portion of the gene that contains exons 1-22 and relocation at considerable distance from the remaining part of the gene, namely, 300 Kb away for inversions that involve the proximal extragenic copy and 400 Kb away when recombination event involves the distal copy (Lakich et al., 1993; Naylor et al., 1995). Thus, transcription from the Factor VIII promoter is possible but a full-length transcript cannot be obtained.

These events occur exclusively during male meiosis, as the X chromosome does not pair with the Y chromosome except at the pseudoautosomal regions, providing ample opportunities for intrachromosomal homologous recombination. This means that the mutation occurs exclusively in the male germline (Becker et al., 1996; Arnheim & Calabrese, 2009), resulting in carrier females born to a healthy mother and a father who carries a germline inversion mutation. Consequently, in the majority of cases where inversion is ultimately found, the haemophilic male who presents at the genetic counseling office is the first case in a family without history for bleeding diathesis. Nevertheless, it is very likely (over 90 %) for a woman who has had one haemophilic son with inversion to be a carrier (Rossiter et al., 1994), therefore the risk of her having another boy affected by haemophilia is close to 50 %, which equals the risk for proven carriers. Explaining to the family the origin of causative mutation and the associated risks could be challenging, especially in the light of the popular notion that women are solely responsible for transmission of haemophilia (as they give birth to affected sons). Generally, about 20-25 % of the females who have had a son with haemophilia have inherited the defective X chromosome from their healthy fathers (Haldane, 1935). Having more than one affected son does not confirm the carrier status of female as the de novo mutation rate in the female germline is estimated to be about 4 times lower than in the male germline (Becker et al.,1996) but is still significant, about 5 %. Of course, for the purposes of prenatal diagnosis 95 % risk of carriership is as good (in the case

of risk assessment, as bad) as 100 %, but nevertheless the genetic counselor must attempt to relieve the psychological burden of female carriership of haemophilia by emphasizing that in terms of de novo mutation occurrence it affects males and females alike, and that inversions occur in males several times more often than in females.

When inversion is the case, the constitution of the disease phenotype could be fairly straightforward. As a rule, inversions of any type (involving distal, proximal and additional copies of the 9.5 Kb repeated unit) result in severe haemophilia with FVIII: C level below 1%, unless another genetic component plays a role (e.g. co-inherited prothrombotic mutations). There are exceptions to the rule but they are fairly infrequent.

It is very important to let parents know exactly what 'severe' means and what potential adverse outcomes there might be. A fairly common parental reaction is overprotectiveness. For chronically ill people of any age, and especially in children, overprotectiveness might actually be of a disadvantage as it might delay the development of various important skills. While parental concern is of prime importance in children with haemophilia, overprotectiveness may actually cause disregard for the major issue in severe haemophilia, namely, the proneness to spontaneous bleeding. Every day, dozens of small-scale bleeding events in the human body trigger the coagulation cascade. Some of them have the potential to develop into life-threatening internal bleedings if coagulation is defective. In haemophiliacs with very low levels of circulating factor bleeding might be provoked by seemingly minor causes or without identifiable reason. Therefore, while overly concerned parents do not let their boy participate insporting activities or play with other children out of fear that it might spiral into a rough-and-tumble that might induce bleeding; they might overlook the importance of checking regularly for signs and symptoms of bleeding. In our practice we had two very caring and protective mothers who, nevertheless, lost their sons following spontaneous bleeding incidents which were not recognized and treated properly because the mothers thought that since there was no preceding traumatic event, there was no cause to worry. It is vital to instill into the family the idea that bleeding must be ruled out first as a reason for any unusual event or complaint in a haemophilic male.

There are other unhealthy psychological states in parents of chronically ill children, including children with haemophilia, that the genetic counselor must recognize and try to intervene. Among these, denial is prominent as it might lead to severe adverse consequences. Denial is often observed in families with young children that have just received diagnosis. Usually, denial in families with haemophilia manifests as unwillingness to accept the fact that the child would not 'outgrow' the disease and avoidance of routine therapy, such as refusing transfusion therapy with Factor VIII preparations and turning to purely symptomatic (cold pads, etc.) or alternative therapies, such as homeopathy, magnet therapy, etc. Unfortunately, parents in denial do not realize that they are paving their child's way for major health trouble. It is the genetic counselor's job to explain that the nature of the molecular defect causing the condition does not allow for the course of the disease to get any better so as to discourage any adverse health practices.

The question of whether immunological response would be launched against the exogenous Factor VIII is more difficult to answer. In cases of inversions with breakpoints within the intron 22 repeated unit, the inversion disrupts the gene structure, precludes generation of a contiguous full-length transcript and results in undetectably low levels of Factor VIII in the patient's plasma. Authors elsewhere have reported relatively high incidence of inhibitor formation in patients with inversion, up to 50 % (Oldenburg et al., 2002; Astermark et al., 2005; Salviato et al., 2007). This is not unusual, as since there is no endogenous synthesis of a

certain protein, any encounter with it might trigger an immune reaction. Surprisingly, however, in our cohort of patients, none of the 25 patients with inversion with breakpoints within the repeated unit in intron 22 developed inhibitors to Factor VIII. This could be explained, however, by the prevailing practice of 'on-demand' treatment, that is, Factor VIII is administered only if there is an evidence of bleeding. Patients and their families should be informed about alternative approaches to combating the immune response to exogenous clotting factors, such as Factor VIIa, as this may generate and/or maintain the motivation for getting adequate treatment.

2.3.2 Point mutations

Generally, nonsense mutations cause premature arrest in mRNA translation, resulting in production of truncated protein. Since factor VIII is a large molecule with a multitude of sites responsible for interaction with other molecules, it is logical to assume that truncated protein variants would have limited, if any, ability to fulfill its functions. Therefore, nonsense mutations usually produce severe haemophilia, unless modulated by additional factors. For such patients, the basic assumptions for counseling families with severe haemophilia stand in place.

Oftentimes non-inversion patients with factor VIII levels below 1 % develop inhibitors, which might be the phenotypic reflection of the immunogenicity of the truncated protein. We have had two patients with severe haemophilia and mutations in the 5' - regulatory region of the Factor VIII gene which supposedly prevented transcription of the gene. Interestingly, they didn't develop antibodies to exogenous Factor VIII, notwithstanding the fact that they have had over 20 years of treatment at the time of referral.

As for missense mutations, it is very much up to the nature of the mutation in question whether the disease would be severe, moderate or mild and it is exactly with missense mutations where other factors (including genetic factors) play the most important role, as the modified protein may lose sites for interaction with other proteins or may, alternatively, gain such sites. As a rule, missense mutations cause CRM-positive haemophilia A with varying severity, depending on the mutation in question and the parts of the gene it affects. Recently, Wakabayashi et al. demonstrated that Factor VIII devoid of its C2 domain remains functional, at least in vitro, but is less stable (Wakabayashi et al., 2010). In our practice, we have had two (related) patients with exon 24 missense mutation (the C2 domain) and with mild haemophilia A (40 %), supporting the notion of decreased stability of the protein.

In moderate haemophilia, prognostication about the course of the disease in the particular patient could be rather difficult and could require a lot of cooperation from the patients and their families so as to carry out all necessary tests that could prompt as to how the defect in the Factor VIII gene clicks in place with other genetic and/or immunological factors that constitute the patient's phenotype. For an example, we have had one adult patient with mild haemophilia according to Factor VIII levels (7 %) but prone since childhood to accidental haematuria without anaemia and/or haemolysis. Since haematuria is not very common even in severe haemophilia, further investigation was undertaken, resulting in identification of co-inherited Factor XI deficiency, as described in Berg et al., (1994). The patient visited the genetic counseling unit so as to get an estimate of risks for transmitting his bleeding tendency to his children (specifically, his newborn daughter) and was, on the one hand, very relieved to know that haemophilia rarely is symptomatic in females, but, on the other, rather discontented to know that there might actually be increased risk of bleeding diathesis.

It could be hard to predict whether the patient would develop antibodies to exogenous Factor VIII in moderate and mild haemophilia. The rule of thumb is, however, that mild haemophilia usually is uneventful in regard to antibody production (in which the less frequent encounter with the exogenous factor preparations may play a role). As for moderate haemophilia, it is advisable that the parents keep a log of the amounts of preparations of clotting factor their child have had, the frequency of infusions and of any adverse events that may occur during or after transfusion so as not to miss the early signs of an impending immune conflict.

2.4 Co-inheritance of prothrombotic mutations

Carriership of molecular defects in other genes coding for proteins acting in the coagulation cascade may produce the so-called "thrombotic phenotype", that is, increased tendency for thrombus formation. Usually, heterozygous carriership of such mutations (also called prothrombotic factors) in healthy people increases the risk of thromboembolism about 2-10 times, depending on the mutation in question (Cumming et al., 1997; Hessner et al., 1999). Homozygous carriership may increase the risk for thrombotic incidents up to 50 - 100-fold (Souto et al., 1999; Ornstein & Cushman, 2003).

The most commonly encountered prothrombotic mutations are the C677T in the 5, 10-methylenetetrahydropholate reductase (MTHFR) gene (very common, prevalence of heterozygous carriership about 30-45 % in the general population), the G1691A substitution in factor V (Factor V Leiden) (between 2 and 6 % in the general population) and the G20210A mutation in the prothrombin gene (2-3 % in the general population) (Cumming et al., 1997; Antoniadi et al., 1999; den Heijer et al., 2003). Generally, about half of the patients with thrombophilia carry either the Factor V Leiden mutation or the G20210 prothrombin mutation (Lillicrap, 1999). Carriership of both mutations in the heterozygous state additionally increases the risk of recurrent thrombosis about three times than the risk for carriers of each mutation alone (De Stefano et al., 1999).

It is believed that the bleeding phenotype in patients with haemophilia might be modulated by concurrent inheritance of prothrombotic risk factors. Indeed, clinical practice often sees patients with clinical course less severe that could be expected from the residual levels of the deficient factor (Escuriola Ettinghausen et al., 2001; Tizzano et al., 2002; Franchini & Lippi, 2010). In such patients the first symptomatic bleeding seems to occur at later age than in haemophilic counterparts without prothrombotic risk factors and the average amount of units per kg body weight used to manage the basic condition is lower. On the other hand, there are reports that co-inheritance of a mutation which causes increased tendency to bleed and a mutation that increases the proneness to thromboembolism may complicate the substitution therapy for haemophilia because of risk of deep venous thrombosis and/or central venous catheter (CVC)-thrombosis during transfusion of Factor VIII-containing preparations (Olcay et al., 1997; Kapur et al., 1997; Ettingshausen et al., 1999).

Therefore, information about the patient's status with regard to most common prothrombotic mutations may increase the degree of confidence when outlining the putative disease phenotype while, at the same time, advise caution when transfusing clotting factor preparations (especially concentrates) to a patient carrying a Factor VIII or factor IX mutation and a prothrombotic risk factor.

2.4.1 Factor V leiden

The process of haemostasis is controlled at numerous levels so as to avoid unmanageable intravasal coagulation. Normally, one of the basic mechanisms to control the clotting

process is proteolytic deactivation of the activated Factor V by activated protein C (APC), a serine protease with anticoagulant properties (Esmon, 1992).

Factor V Leiden (FVL) is a common mutation in the factor V gene resulting in thrombophilia [Bertina et al., 1994]. The factor V protein product bears a high degree of homology to Factor VIII - both in domain structure and in function, as Factor V acts as a cofactor of factor Xa in the coagulation cascade (Kane & Davie, 1988). The Factor V gene, however, is an autosomal gene. In their homozygous state, mutation events disrupting the Factor V gene cause a rare bleeding diathesis called parahaemophilia or Owren's disease (Owren, 1947).

The Factor V Leiden mutation is a G→A transition at nucleotide 1691 in exon 10 of the Factor V gene. At protein level this produces an Arg-to-Gln substitution which renders Factor V molecule uncleavable by APC, therefore resistant to its anticoagulant action. In healthy people this usually increases the risk for deep venous thromboses (DVTs) - mainly in the veins of the legs, but but also in the veins of the arms, the lungs, the abdomen, and the brain. In pregnant women, carriership of Factor V Leiden (and other prothrombotic mutations) is associated with multiplying (between 10 and 15-fold) the risk for of venous thromboembolism during pregnancy and late fetal loss (Koeleman et al., 1994; Gerhardt et al., 2000, Martinelli et al., 2000). When co-inherited with haemophilia, FVL may modulate the bleeding phenotype and/or complicate the therapy with coagulation factor preparations.

2.4.2 Prothrombin G20210A mutation

The prothrombin-thrombin conversion is a key step in the coagulation cascade. The prothrombin G20210A variant (PT20210) is the second most common genetic mutation enhancing blood clotting. Again, it is autosomally inherited and is a transition G→A but it has no effect on the coding sequence of the encoded protein, rather, it affects the polyadenylation site in the prothrombin gene (Poort et al., 1996), causing increased prothrombin levels in plasma. As with Factor V Leiden, the carriership of the PT20210 mutation results in increased risk for thrombotic events (Chamouard et al., 1999; Franco et al., 2009), associated with the same concerns in patients with haemophilia who are on replacement therapy.

2.4.3 MTHFR C677T mutation

The human gene for 5,10-methylenetetrahydrofolate reductase is an autosomal gene coding for an enzyme catalyzing the conversion of 5,10-methylenetetrahydrofolate to 5-methyltetrahydrofolate (Goyette et al., 1994), the latter being a substrate for methionine synthase catalyzing the homocysteine remethylation to methionine. The mutation is a C→T transition in the protein coding regions of the gene, causing an alanine to valine substitution in exon 4 and reduced enzyme activity (Frosst et al., 1995). The resulting phenotype is of homocysteinemia associated with increased risk of vascular disease and thrombosis.

The prevalence of the C677T mutation is very high in all ethnic groups. The heterozygous (CT) state is seen in 20 to 50 % in different populations while the TT homozygotes may amount up to 30 % (Wilcken et al., 2003), hence, it would certainly co-occur with haemophilia in a significant proportion of the patients.

Since the prothrombotic mutations predispose to increased tendency for blood clotting, presumably co-inheritance of prothrombotic mutations and a mutation in the Factor VIII or Factor IX genes causing haemophilia might result in amelioration of the disease phenotype. This could present as later age of onset (age at which first symptomatic

bleeding occurs - for severe haemophilia typically around the age of 9-12 months when the baby learns to walk and bumps and falls are frequent) and/or fewer serious bleeding episodes and/or less episodes of spontaneous bleeding and/or less frequent rebleeding (rebleeding is a fairly frequent occurrence in haemophilia patients, as the clot, when finally formed, is friable and prone to breaking apart) and/or use of less units of the deficient clotting factor (Lee et al., 2000).

The flip side of the coin in co-inheritance of common prothrombotic mutations and haemophilia is the risk for complications of therapy, related to the fact that the presence of the prothrombotic mutation often increases the rate of thrombin formation (van 't Veer et al., 1997). The several hundreds or thousands of coagulation factor units needed to stabilize the patient's haemostasis are often transfused rapidly, within one minute or even faster. The general recommendation is that any blood clotting factor preparation should be infused slowly with no more than 2 ml of solution infused per minute so as to avoid complications, but the unfortunate practice shows that in at-home treatment schemes and sometimes even in clinical settings the whole amount of 3-10 ml of reconstituted coagulation factor is infused too rapidly - within a couple of dozens of seconds, out of desire to achieve results faster. Thus, in haemophilic patients with prothrombotic mutations, the therapy with clotting factors may provoke thromboembolic events - with disastrous consequences for the patient. There have been reports of cerebral and cardiac thrombotic incidents associated with Factor V Leiden carriership in haemophilic patients (Olcay et al., 1997, Iannaccaro et al., 2005). Therefore, it is important to screen haemophilic patients for prothrombotic mutations - with regard to possible disease phenotype modulation as well as in relation to possible modifications of therapy, in order to prevent adverse events.

Our experience to date shows that the three most common prothrombotic mutations (Factor V Leiden, PT20210 and MTHFR C677T) seem not to modulate the disease phenotype in all patients with haemophilia. Apparently, Bulgarian patients with severe haemophilia gain no benefits from neither of the co-inherited prothrombotic mutations, as all identified carriers exhibit the classical 'severe' phenotype, with frequent spontaneous bleedings and age of onset before the first year of life. There was no difference between the number of haemorrhagic episodes and/or the units of Factor VIII used per kg body weight per year between patients carrying prothrombotic mutations and patients who did not have additional mutations affecting components of blood coagulation cascade. It seems that the carriership of prothrombotic mutations does not contribute to the phenotype constitution in the local haemophilic population.

It could be challenging to predict whether and when in the course of therapy a haemophilic patient might experience a thrombotic event, especially if the patient is very young at the time of referral. Considering the risks that are associated with replacement therapy, however, it is advisable that the families are warned about the possibility of thromboembolism during or after clotting factor application. Until proven otherwise, identification of a prothrombotic mutation in a patient with severe haemophilia is another factor that should be considered as an additional potential risk source when defining the risks associated with therapy. It is vital to teach the family members that in case of signs of impending haemorrhage quick action is advisable but that speed should be made in contacting the attending physician (if deemed necessary), obtaining the clotting factor preparation (if it is not immediately available) and preparing it for use but not in the process of infusion itself as it may lead to severe adverse events. Patients with non-00 AB0 blood group should constitute a group of special concern for such events as it has been repeatedly

demonstrated that blood group different from 00 additionally increases the risk for thrombosis about 5-fold (Fontcuberta et al., 2008; Jukic et al., 2009).

In our practice we have observed patients with Haemophilia A and unusually mild bleeding phenotype discordant with the level of residual factor - 0-1 % as determined by at least two independent tests. Namely, the patients were seldom treated with factor VIII - less than six times per year - usually as a preventative measure before surgery or dental procedures. Bleeding incidents were usually preceded by a precipitating event and managed effectively by bandaging, cold applications and rest. Only one patient (55 years of age at time of referral) had unilateral haemophilic arthropathy of the knee which did not interfere significantly with everyday activities. Interestingly, in about half of these patients the causative mutation of the factor VIII gene was the large inversion involving the repeated unit in intron 22, therefore, the milder phenotype could not be explained by Factor VIII-gene related reasons (in-frame deletions, 'leaky' mutations, etc). None of these patients had a Factor V Leiden or PTG20210 mutation and the prevalence of MTHFR C677T in this group did not differ significantly from the basic values for European Caucasoid populations (30 %). It is possible that the milder phenotype might be attributed to carriership of MTHFR C677T but, as of now, until proven otherwise, carriership of any prothrombotic mutation must be considered to be associated with increased risk for adverse effects of the replacement therapy. Families should be advised to keep a log of the infused units and the frequency of infusions of clotting factor-containing preparations so as to illuminate any positive connection between co-carriership of prothrombotic mutations and milder course in haemophilia.

Women carriers of prothrombotic mutations are at risk of preeclampsia and fetal loss. Female carriers of haemophilia and prothrombotic mutations who are pregnant or planning to become pregnant should be informed about the risks associated with the pregnancy (risks for having a haemophilic boy stemming from the carriership of haemophilia-producing mutation and risks for both the mother and the foetus because of the carriership of a prothrombotic mutation) and referred for intensive pregnancy monitoring so as to avoid complications. Again, contribution of other risk-modifying factors such as AB0 blood group, smoking, etc. should be evaluated.

2.5 Infections transmitted by transfusion of blood or blood products

The risk of infection with any of the common blood-transmitted diseases is significant for patients receiving regular transfusions of plasma, blood and blood products. Even considering the improvements in the sensitivity of the methods screening for infectious disease transmitted by blood and blood products, there still remains a risk for infection which is proportional to the number of occasions in which the patient has been exposed to blood, plasma, cryoprecipitate, etc. Basically all Bulgarian patients over 20 years of age are chronically Hb_sAg - positive and a significant proportion of them test as HCV-positive. Thankfully, the rates of new infection with blood-transmitted diseases in Bulgarian haemophilic patients is experiencing a steady decline thanks to the introduction of recombinant Factor VIII, IX and VIIa preparations in routine practice.

It is, however, a common concern of families of patients with haemophilia that the replacement treatment may bring about adverse events associated with transmission of infectious agents, which may lead to adverse health practices. This might be especially true for parents with young, newly diagnosed children who are not yet acquainted with the risks of spontaneous bleeding and/or the long-term effects of untreated haemophilia on joints, internal organs and the brain, and also for parents who are in denial. Such parents may

choose not to treat their child or may revert to alternative treatments, believing that the consequences of blood-transmitted diseases might be graver than the consequences of repeated bleedings. Typically, however, refusal of replacement treatment by the parents is not associated with parental neglect but, rather, with overprotectiveness, the behaviour stemming from from the erroneous belief that if parents are watchful enough so as not to allow physical trauma of the child, bleeding would not occur. Also, there might be significant parental opposition to the idea of using recombinant coagulation factor preparations out of fear that this might actually increase the risk of antibody production. It is vital that the attending clinician together with the genetic counselor review all the therapeutic options with the family and and provide reliable information about the rates of infection with blood-transmissive agents when using different coagulation factor preparations. Misconceptions related to the idea that the replacement could actually make the child more ill should be carefully addressed and any associated practices should be actively discouraged.

3. Conclusion

You have to make the good out of the bad
because that is all you have got to make it out of.
Robert Penn Warren, All King's Men (1946)

Haemophilias produce a heterogeneous phenotype which may be modulated by a number of factors, endogenous or resulting from outside intervention. There is a significant inter-patient variety of disease phenotype even in related patients due to the fact that the clinical severity is not always correlated with the residual level of the clotting factor. Genetic counselling for haemophilia is a continuous process which aims at gathering maximal amount of genetic information pertaining to the nature of genetic mutation causing the disease in the particular family, the carriership of additional genetic variants that might modulate the phenotype and the potential risks associated with specific traits in the patient's genetic background. In genetic counselling, the patients, their families, the attending clinicians, the genetic counselling unit and the clinical laboratory specialists ought to work as a team in order to obtain and process information related to the genetic and immunological status of the patient and to come up with a management strategy tailored out specifically to the needs of the patient. Careful weighing of the risks is important when presenting the facts about the familial disease and needless adverse psychological impact related to the grave diagnosis and the risks of further transmission of the disease should be minimized.

The genetic counseling unit should be able to provide answers to the vital questions of the family associated with the well-being of the affected child/ren and the opportunities for family planning. Dealing with popular misconceptions such as the notion that having had one affected son means automatically that the mother is a carrier and the erroneous belief that haemophilia could be eventually outgrown must also be on the to-do list of the genetic counseling unit as the information they present could provide a convincing proof that the disease transmission is governed by strict rules and tends to have a chronic course. It is only through dialogue that the best possible outcome for the patient and for the family is attained; therefore the process of genetic counseling should include asking a lot of questions and giving a lot of answers in order to achieve the optimal results.

4. Acknowledgements

The author/s wish to thank the patients and their families for participating in the studies associated with the present work as well as the attending clinical and laboratory specialists for providing us with the relevant details of the medical history and the laboratory tests. This research was supported by grant No. DO02-69 of the Ministry of Education, Youth and Science of Republic of Bulgaria.

5. References

Aledort LM. Is the incidence and prevalence of inhibitors greater with recombinant products? Yes. J Thromb Haemost. 2004 Jun;2(6):861-2.

Antoniadi T, Hatzis T, Kroupis C, Economou-Petersen E & Petersen MB. Prevalence of factor V Leiden, prothrombin G20210A, and MTHFR C677T mutations in a Greek population of blood donors. Am J Hematol. 1999 Aug;61(4):265-7.

Arnheim N & Calabrese P. Understanding what determines the frequency and pattern of human germline mutations.Nat Rev Genet. 2009 Jul;10(7):478-88.

Astermark J. Inhibitor development: patient-determined risk factors. Haemophilia. 2010 May;16(102):66-70.

Astermark J, Oldenburg J, Escobar M, White GC 2nd, Berntorp E & Malmö International Brother Study study group. The Malmö International Brother Study (MIBS). Genetic defects and inhibitor development in siblings with severe hemophilia A. Haematologica. 2005 Jul;90(7):924-31.

Becker J, Schwaab R, Möller-Taube A, Schwaab U, Schmidt W, Brackmann HH, Grimm T, Olek K & Oldenburg J. Characterization of the factor VIII defect in 147 patients with sporadic hemophilia A: family studies indicate a mutation type-dependent sex ratio of mutation frequencies.Am J Hum Genet. 1996 Apr;58(4):657-70.

Berg LP, Varon D, Martinowitz U, Wieland K, Kakkar VV & Cooper DN. Combined factor VIII/factor XI deficiency may cause intra-familial clinical variability on haemophilia A among Ashkenazi Jews. Blood Coagul Fibrinol 1994; 5: 59-62.

Bertina RM, Koeleman BP, Koster T, Rosendaal FR, Dirven RJ, de Ronde H, van der Velden PA & Reitsma PH. Mutation in blood coagulation factor V associated with resistance to activated protein C. Nature. 1994 May 5;369(6475):64-7.

de Biasi R, Rocino A, Papa ML, Salerno E, Mastrullo L & De Blasi D. Incidence of factor VIII inhibitor development in hemophilia A patients treated with less pure plasma derived concentrates. Thromb Haemost. 1994;7:544–547.

Chamouard P, Pencreach E, Maloisel F, Grunebaum L, Ardizzone JF, Meyer A, Gaub MP, Goetz J, Baumann R, Uring-Lambert B, Levy S, Dufour P, Hauptmann G & Oudet P. Frequent factor II G20210A mutation in idiopathic portal vein thrombosis. Gastroenterology. 1999 Jan;116(1):144-8.

Chaves D, Belisário A, Castro G, Santoro M & Rodrigues C. Analysis of cytokine genes polymorphism as markers for inhibitor development in haemophilia A. Int J Immunogenet. 2010 Apr;37(2):79-82.

Cumming AM, Keeney S, Salden A, Bhavnani M, Shwe KH & Hay CR. The prothrombin gene G20210A variant: prevalence in a U.K. anticoagulant clinic population. Br J Haematol. 1997 Aug;98(2):353-5.

Denson KW. The detection of factor-VIII-like antigen in haemophilic carriers and in patients with raised levels of biologically active factor VIII. Br J Haematol. 1973 Apr;24(4):451-61.

d'Oiron R, Pipe SW & Jacquemin M. Mild/moderate haemophilia A: new insights into molecular mechanisms and inhibitor development. Haemophilia. 2008 Jul;14 Suppl 3:138-46.

Goudemand J, Rothschild C, Demiguel V, Vinciguerrat C, Lambert T, Chambost H, Borel-Derlon A, Claeyssens S, Laurian Y, Calvez T & FVIII-LFB and Recombinant FVIII study groups. Influence of the type of factor VIII concentrate on the incidence of factor VIII inhibitors in previously untreated patients with severe hemophilia A. Blood. 2006;107:46–51.

Escuriola Ettinghausen C, Halimeh S, Kurnik K, Shobess R, Wermes C, Junker R, Kreuz W, Pollmann H & Nowak-Gottl U. Symptomatic onset of severe haemophilia A in childhood is dependent on the presence of prothrombotic risk factors. Thromb and Haemost 2001 Feb ; 85(2): 218-220.

Esmon CT. The protein C anticoagulant pathway. Arterioscler Thromb 1992 Feb;12(2):135-45.

Ettingshausen C, Saguer IM & Kreutz W. Portal vein thrombosis in a patient with severe haemophilia A and F V G1691A mutation during continuous infusion of F VIII after intramural jejunal bleeding-successful thrombolysis under heparin therapy. Eur J Pediatr. 1999 Dec; 158 Suppl 3:S180-2.

Franchini M & Lippi G. Factor V Leiden and hemophilia.Thromb Res. 2010 Feb;125(2):119-23.

Franco RF, Trip MD, ten Cate H, van den Ende A, Prins MH, Kastelein JJ & Reitsma PH. The 20210 G-->A mutation in the 3'-untranslated region of the prothrombin gene and the risk for arterial thrombotic disease. Br J Haematol. 1999 Jan;104(1):50-4.

Frosst P, Blom HJ, Milos R, Goyette P, Sheppard CA, Matthews RG, Boers GJ, den Heijer M, Kluijtmans LA & van den Heuvel LP. A candidate genetic risk factor for vascular disease: a common mutation in methylenetetrahydrofolate reductase. Nat Genet. 1995 May;10(1):111-3.

Gerhardt A, Scharf RE, Beckmann MW, Struve S, Bender HG, Pillny M, Sandmann W & Zotz RB. Prothrombin and factor V mutations in women with a history of thrombosis during pregnancy and the puerperium. N Engl J Med. 2000 Feb 10;342(6):374-80.

Ghosh K & Shetty S. Immune response to FVIII in hemophilia A: an overview of risk factors. Clin Rev Allergy Immunol. 2009 Oct;37(2):58-66.

Gitschier J, Wood W, Goralka T, Wion K, Chen E, Eaton D, Vehar G, Capon D & Lawn R. Characterization of the human factor VIII gene. Nature, vol. 312, 22, Nov 1984.

Goodeve AC & Peake IR. The molecular basis of hemophilia A: genotype-phenotype relationships and inhibitor development. Semin Thromb Hemost. 2003 Feb;29(1):23-30.

Gouw SC, van der Bom JG, Auerswald G, Ettinghausen CE, Tedgard U & van den Berg HM. Recombinant versus plasma-derived factor VIII products and the development of inhibitors in previously untreated patients with severe hemophilia A: The CANAL cohort study. Blood. 2007;109:4693–4697.

Gouw SC, van der Bom JG, van den Berg HM, Zewald RA, Ploos vanAmstel JK & Mauser-Bunschoten EP. Influence of the type of F8 gene mutation on inhibitor development in a single centre cohort of severe haemophilia A patients. Haemophilia. 2011 Mar; 17(2):275-281.

Goyette P, Sumner JS, Milos R, Duncan AM, Rosenblatt DS, Matthews RG & Rozen R. Human methylenetetrahydrofolate reductase: isolation of cDNA, mapping and mutation identification. Nat Genet. 1994 Jun;7(2):195-200.

Hay CR, Ollier W, Pepper L, Cumming A, Keeney S, Goodeve AC, Colvin BT, Hill FG, Preston FE & Peake IR. HLA class II profile: a weak determinant of factor VIII

inhibitor development in severe haemophilia A. UKHCDO Inhibitor Working Party.Thromb Haemost. 1997 Feb;77(2):234-7.

den Heijer M, Lewington S & Clarke R. Homocysteine, MTHFR and risk of venous thrombosis: a meta-analysis of published epidemiological studies. J Thromb Haemost 2005;3: 292-9.

Hessner MJ, Luhm RA, Pearson SL, Endean DJ, Friedman KD & Montgomery RR. Prevalence of prothrombin G20210A, factor V G1691A (Leiden), and methylenetetrahydrofolate reductase (MTHFR) C677T in seven different populations determined by multiplex allele-specific PCR. Thromb Haemost. 1999 May;81(5):733-8.

Iannaccaro P, Santoro R, Sottilotta G, Papaleo G & Muleo G. Thrombosis in hemophiliacs with prothrombotic molecular defect. Clin Appl Thromb Hemost. 2005 Jul;11(3):359-60.

Jukic I, Bingulac-Popovic J, Dogic V, Babic I, Culej J, Tomicic M, Vuk T, Sarlija D & Balija M. ABO blood groups and genetic risk factors for thrombosis in Croatian population. Croat Med J. 2009 Dec;50(6):550-8.

Kane WH & Davie EW. Blood coagulation factors V and VIII: structural and functional similarities and their relationship to haemorrhagic and thrombotic disorders. 1988, Blood, 71: 539-55.

Kapur RK, Mills LA, Spitzer SG & Hultin MB. A prothrombin gene mutation is significantly associated with venous thrombosis. Arterioscler Thromb Vasc Biol. 1997 Nov;17(11):2875-9.

Kazazian HH, Tuddenham EGD & Antonarakis SE. (1995). Hemophilia A and parahemophilia : deficiencies of coagulation factors VIII and V. In: The Metabolic and Molecular Bases of Inherited Disease, 8th ed. Scriver CR, Beaudet A, Valle D & Sly W. (eds). pp. (3241-3267). McGraw-Hill Professional, ISBN-10 0079130356, New York City, USA.

Koeleman BPC, Reitsma PH, Allaart CF, Bertina RM. Activated protein C resistance as an additional risk factor for thrombosis in protein C-deficient families. Blood 84: 1031-1035, 1994.

Lakich D, Kazazian H Jr., Antonarakis S & Gitschier J. Inversions disrupting the factor VIII gene are a common cause of severe haemophilia A. Nature Genetics, vol. 5, Nov 1993.

Lee DH, Walker IR, Teitel J, Poon MC, Ritchie B, Akabutu J, Sinclair GD, Pai M, Wu JW, Reddy S, Carter C, Growe G, Lillicrap D, Lam M & Blajchman MA. Effect of the factor V Leiden mutation on the clinical expression of severe hemophilia A. Thromb Haemost. 2000 Mar;83(3):387-91.

Levinson, B., Kenwrick, S., Lakich, D., Hammonds, G. Jr, & Gitschier, J. A transcribed gene in an intron of the human factor VIII gene. Genomics. 1990 May; 7(1):1-11.

Levinson B, Kenwrick S, Gamel P, Fisher K, & Gitschier J. Evidence for a third transcript from the human factor VIII gene. 1992, Genomics, 14, 585-589.

Lillicrap D. Molecular diagnosis of inherited bleeding disorders and thrombophilia. Semin Haematol 1999 Oct; 36 (4): 340-351.

Margaglione M, Castaman G, Morfini M, Rocino A, Santagostino E, Tagariello G, Tagliaferri AR, Zanon E, Bicocchi MP, Castaldo G, Peyvandi F, Santacroce R, Torricelli F, Grandone E, Mannucci PM & AICE-Genetics Study Group. The Italian AICE-Genetics hemophilia A database: results and correlation with clinical phenotype. Haematologica. 2008 May;93(5):722-8.

Martinelli I, Taioli E, Cetin I, Marinoni A, Gerosa S, Villa MV, Bozzo M & Mannucci PM. Mutations in coagulation factors in women with unexplained late fetal loss. N Engl J Med. 2000 Oct 5;343(14):1015-8.

Miñano A, Ordóñez A, España F, González-Porras JR, Lecumberri R, Fontcuberta J, Llamas P, Marín F, Estellés A, Alberca I, Vicente V & Corral J. AB0 blood group and risk of venous or arterial thrombosis in carriers of factor V Leiden or prothrombin G20210A polymorphisms. Haematologica. 2008 May;93(5):729-34.

Naylor JA, Brinke A, Hassock S, Green PM & Giannelli F. Characteristic mRNA abnormality found in half the patients with severe haemophilia A is due to large DNA inversions. Hum Mol Genet, 1993; 2: 1773-1778.

Naylor J, Buck D, Green P, Williamson H, Bentley D, Giannelli F. Investigation of the Factor VII repeated region (int22h) and the associated inversion junctions. Hum Mol Genet 1995; vol. 4, No 7.

Olcay L, Gurgey A, Topaloglu H, Altay S, Parlak H & Firat M. Cerebral infarct associated with factor V Leiden mutation in a boy with haemophilia A. Am J Haematol 1997; Nov, 56(3): 189-90.

Oldenburg J, El-Maarri O & Schwaab R. Inhibitor development in correlation to factor VIII genotypes. Haemophilia. 2002 Mar;8 Suppl 2:23-9.

Oldenburg J, Brackmann HH & Schwaab R. Risk factors for inhibitor development in hemophilia A. Haematologica. 2000;85:7–13.

Ornstein DL & Cushman M. Factor V Leiden. Circulation. 2003;107:e94.

Owren P. Parahaemophilia: haemorrhagic diathesis due to absence of a previously unknown clotting factor. Lancet 249: 446-448, 1947.

Pavlova A, Delev D, Lacroix-Desmazes S, Schwaab R, Mende M, Fimmers R, Astermark J & Oldenburg J. Impact of polymorphisms of the major histocompatibility complex class II, interleukin-10, tumor necrosis factor-alpha and cytotoxic T-lymphocyte antigen-4 genes on inhibitor development in severe hemophilia A. J Thromb Haemost. 2009 Dec;7(12):2006-2015.

Pittman DD, Milenson M, Marquette K, Bauer K & Kaufman RJ. A2 domain of human recombinant derived factor VIII is required for procoagulant activity but not for thrombin cleavage. Blood 1992; Jan 15; 79:2, 389-97.

Poort SR, Rosendaal FR, Reitsma PH & Bertina RM. A common genetic variation in the 3'-untranslated region of the prothrombin gene is associated with elevated plasma prothrombin levels and an increase in venous thrombosis.Blood. 1996 Nov 15;88(10):3698-703.

Ragni MV, Ojeifo O, Feng J, Yan J, Hill KA, Sommer SS, Trucco MN, Brambilla DJ & Hemophilia Inhibitor Study. Risk factors for inhibitor formation in haemophilia: a prevalent case-control study. Haemophilia. 2009 Sep;15(5):1074-82.

Reiner P & Thompson AR. Screening for nonsense mutations in patients with severe haemophilia A can provide rapid, direct carrier detection. Hum Genet (1992) 89:88-94.

Roberts HR, Grizzle JE, McLester WD & Penick GO. Genetic variants of haemophilia B. Detection by means of a specific PTC inhibitor. J Clin Invest 1968, 47:360.

Rossiter JP, Young M, Kimberland ML, Hutter P, Ketterling RP, Gitschier J, Horst J, Morris MA, Schaid DJ & De Moerloose P. Factor VIII gene causing severe haemophilia A inversions originate almost exclusively in male germ cells. 1994, Hum Mol Genet, 3: 1035-39.

Salviato R, Belvini D, Radossi P, Sartori R, Pierobon F, Zanotto D, Zanon E, Castaman G, Gandini G & Tagariello G. F8 gene mutation profile and ITT response in a cohort of Italian haemophilia A patients with inhibitors. Haemophilia. 2007 Jul;13(4):361-72.

Souto JC, Mateo J, Soria JM, Llobet D, Coll I, Borrell M & Fontcuberta J (1999). Homozygotes for prothrombin gene 20210 A allele in a thrombophilic family without clinical manifestations of venous thromboembolism. Haematologica, 84(7), 627-632.

Schwaab R, Brackmann HH, Meyer C, Seehafer J, Kirchgesser M, Haack A, Olek K,

Tuddenham EG, Cooper DN, Gitschier J, Higuchi M, Hoyer LW, Yoshioka A, Peake IR, Schwaab R, Olek K & Kazazian HH. Haemophilia A: database of nucleotide substitutions, deletions, insertions and rearrangements of the factor VIII gene. Nucleic Acids Res. 1991 Sep 25;19(18):4821-33.

De Stefano V, Martinelli I, Mannucci PM, Paciaroni K, Chiusolo P, Casorelli I, Rossi E & Leone G. The risk of recurrent deep venous thrombosis among heterozygous carriers of both factor V Leiden and the G20210A prothrombin mutation. N Engl J Med. 1999 Sep 9;341(11):801-6.

Tizzano EF, Soria JM, Coll I, Guzman B, Cornet M, Altisent C, Martorell M, Domenech M, del Rio E, Fontcuberta J & Baiget M. The prothrombin 20210 allele influences clinical manifestations of hemophila A in patients with intron 22 inversion and without inhibitors. Haematologica 2002; Mar, 87(3): 279-85.

Tuddenham EGD, Schwaab R, Seehafer J, Millar DS, Gitschier J, Higuchi M, Bidichandani S, Connor JM, Hoyer LW, Yoshioka A, Peake IR, Olek K, Kazazian HH, Lavergne J-M, Giannelli F, Antonarakis SE & Cooper DN. Haemophilia A: database of nucleotide substitutions, deletions, insertions and rearrangements of the factor VIII gene, second edition. Nucleic Acids Res 1994; 22: 4851-4868.

Tuddenham EG & Oldenburg J. Haemophilia A: mutation type determines risk of inhibitor formation. Thromb Haemost. 1995 Dec;74(6):1402-6.

van 't Veer C, Golden NJ, Kalafatis M, Simioni P, Bertina RM & Mann KG. An in vitro analysis of the combination of hemophilia A and factor V(LEIDEN). Blood. 1997 Oct 15;90(8):3067-72.

Wakabayashi H & Fay PJ. Identification of residues contributing to A2 domain-dependent structural stability in factor VIII and factor VIIIa. J Biol Chem. 2008 Apr 25;283(17):11645-51.

Wakabayashi H, Griffiths AE & Fay PJ. Factor VIII lacking the C2 domain retains cofactor activity in vitro.J Biol Chem. 2010 Aug 13;285(33):25176-84.

Wilcken B, Bamforth F, Li Z, Zhu H, Ritvanen A, Renlund M, Stoll C, Alembik Y, Dott B, Czeizel AE, Gelman-Kohan Z, Scarano G, Bianca S, Ettore G, Tenconi R, Bellato S, Scala I, Mutchinick OM, López MA, de Walle H, Hofstra R, Joutchenko L, Kavteladze L, Bermejo E, Martínez-Frías ML, Gallagher M, Erickson JD, Vollset SE, Mastroiacovo P, Andria G & Botto LD. Geographical and ethnic variation of the 677C>T allele of 5,10 ethylenetetrahydrofolate reductase (MTHFR): findings from over 7000 newborns from 16 areas worldwide. J Med Genet. 2003 Aug;40(8):619-25.

Youssoffian H, Kazazian HH, Phillips DG, Aronis S, Tsiftis G, Brown VA & Antonarakis SE. Recurrent mutations in haemophilia A give evidence for CpG mutation hotspots. 1986; Nature 324:380-382.

Youssouffian H, Antonarakis SE, Aronis S, Triftis G, Phillipis DG, & Kazazian HH Jr. Characterization of five partial deletions of the factor VIII gene. Proc Natl Acad Sci USA 1987, 84:3772.

Zimmermann TS & Edgington TS. Factor VIII coagulant activity and factor VIII like antigen : Independent molecular entities. J Exp Med 1973, 138: 1015.

4

Population Evolution in Hemophilia

Myung-Hoon Chung
Hongik University, Jochiwon
Korea

1. Introduction

Gene defects cause diseases. It is reasonable to argue that a disease is related to many genes and a gene affects on many diseases. This multiple-to-multiple mapping between genes and diseases makes it difficult to understand the roles of genes completely. However, in some case, only one gene is involved in one disease. A good example of one-to-one mapping is hemophilia related to gene F8 (National Hemophilia Foundation, 1998).

Biologists found that there are approximately 3 billion nitrogenous bases in 44+2 human DNA. Most sequences of these bases are irrelevant to genetic inheritance. Less than 3% of whole pair sequences are known to determine characteristic features of all human genes (Lander et al., 2001; Venter et al., 2001). Since the diversity of human's inherited characteristics is huge, it can only be explained by cooperation of multiple genes.

Single gene effect with multiple alleles such as blood groups (Chung et al., 1997), color blindness and hemophilia (Lee et al., 2001) can be studied by using the automata equations. Their solutions have some analogy with fixed points of renormalization group equations in physics (Mekjian, 1991; Perelson & Weisbuch, 1997), and lead into the Hardy-Weinberg formula (Haldane, 1935; Hedrick, 1985; Li, 1976).

We extended the automata equations to investigate multiple gene effects on population evolution with any number of loci and alleles in the presence of mutation and selection (Chung et al., 2003). As results of the study, we present the generalized Hardy-Weinberg formula and a simulation program on the Internet (Chung, 2007). The program explores simultaneous control of parameters that affect the behavior of gene variations in a population. We note that Hampe *et al.* (1998) studied population evolution in a different view point from ours. The advantage of our approach is that we do not need a large RAM memory because we do not treat individual person, but consider groups characterized by genes. One more good point beyond the work of Hampe *et al.* (1998) is that we achieve quickly equilibrium state. Using the simulation program, we find that the mortality rates due to gene inheritance are greatly enhanced for multiple gene cases. Another user friendly simulation program provides a convenient scheme for the most common cases (Quardokus, 2000). However, it is not easy to extend this scheme to include more sophisticated situations.

Human beings inherit not only biological genes but also social status from their parents. A few examples of the social inheritance are family name, nationality, or wealth. One of the outstanding questions is how or whether this social inheritance influences the standard biological gene evolution. We believe that this type of interaction may play a crucial

role in explaining appearance or disappearance of certain physical or social traits in some communities. In order to study population evolution with inheritance of social status, we treat inheritable social traits as *social genes* that behave similar to Mendelian genes. This approach allows us to handle the biological and the social genes in a unified way and to examine the mutual influence between the social and the biological genes.

One of the distinct features of the social gene is that it causes preferential non-random mating. Non-random mating exists even without the social gene concepts. Desire to avoid genetically inherited diseases and preferential sexual attraction may cause non-random mating. However, with the social restriction and prejudice, the tendency of non-random mating is expected to become more prominent and complicated.

The population evolution depends on four dominant factors imposed by nature with genes. These factors are (1) mating, (2) mutation, (3) reproduction, and (4) selection. The author proposed automata equations in order to describe the effects of these factors in the population evolution. These equations were used to determine the equilibrium population ratios in multiple gene inheritance, where arbitrary numbers of loci and alleles were allowed in the presence of natural selection, mutation and recombination. A user-friendly numerical simulation program was proposed for estimation of the infant mortality rate for fatal diseases (Chung et al., 2003). In order to incorporate the social genes in the inheritance scheme, we generalize the scheme to include non-random mating explicitly.

It is worthwhile to mention other population evolution studies, which are different from our approach. First of all, Cavalli-Sforza and Feldman (1981) developed a mathematically-rich theory of cultural transmission and evolution. Gene-culture coevolution refers to the evolutionary phenomena that arise from interactions between the biological and social inheritance systems (Aoki, 2001). In genetics, there exist current efforts to locate genes that contribute to diseases or to valuable traits (Piccolboni & Gusfield, 2003). Furthermore, it is essential to analyze the structure of populations on the basis of genetic data (Santafe et al., 2008). It is also well-known that the coalescent method (Hudson, 1991) is use to determine mutation rates (Thomson et al., 2000) and recombination rates (Fu & Li, 1999) in the way of statistical inference (Rosenberg & Nordborg, 2002). Studies on substructured populations introduce the similar feature of social gene, for instance, age (Charlesworth, 1994) or last name. We note that many studies related to mating already exist. The convergence of the multilocus systems under selection with a random mating was investigated (Nagylaki et al., 1999). In the population models for the diploid ancestral process with a random mating, the convergence criterium was proved (Möhle et al., 2003). Non-random mating has been found to play a significant role in the models of the population genetics. In the work related with a non-random mating (Hausken & Hirshleifer, 2001), the truthful signalling hypothesis was used in the mating competition theory. Strategic mating between males and females was also considered by Alpern and Reyniers (2005) and Radcliffe and Rass (1999).

The main purpose of this chapter is to provide a theoretical scheme and a simulation tool to handle the social and the biological genes in a unified way. We present a generalized numerical simulation tool to account for the role of the non-random mating induced by the social genes in addition to mutation, recombination and selection. We expect that the scheme will allow one to examine closely the impact of the social genes on the biological ones and vice versa. For example, we study hemophilia thoroughly without and with a social gene. Simulation results show that a medical screening to prevent birth of females with fatal

hemophilia increases the number of the male patients and the female carriers, thus clearly showing that the social effects significantly influence the inheritance of the biological gene.

2. Model

2.1 Symbols

The fundamental concept for the population evolution is the gene, which allows multiple loci, multiple allele inheritance with recombination and mutation. The l-th gene in the i-th chromosome is labeled by two indices (i, l). We denote $n^{(i,l)}$ as the number of alleles for the gene. Hence, we denote gene

$$G_a^{(i,l)},$$

where $1 \leq a \leq n^{(i,l)}$ and $i = 1, 2, \cdots, 22, X, Y, m, s$ including sex chromosome X, Y, mitochondria m, and social gene s. Here, we note that the social inheritance is treated on an equal footing with the biological one. However, the social genes may have different rules of reproduction and mutation rates, when compared with the biological genes.

The string of genes models each chromosome. We denote chromosome $C_a^{(i)}$ containing relevant L_i genes as

$$C_a^{(i)} = G_{a_1}^{(i,1)} G_{a_2}^{(i,2)} \cdots G_{a_{L_i}}^{(i,L_i)},$$

with $i = 1, 2, \cdots, 22, X, Y$. We write mitochondria M_a containing relevant L_m genes as

$$M_a = G_{a_1}^{(m,1)} G_{a_2}^{(m,2)} \cdots G_{a_{Lm}}^{(m,L_m)}.$$

Also we write social gene string S_a containing relevant L_s genes as

$$S_a = G_{a_1}^{(s,1)} : G_{a_2}^{(s,2)} : \cdots : G_{a_{L_s}}^{(s,L_s)}.$$

The number of distinguishable strings is given by $\prod_{l=1}^{L_i} n^{(i,l)} \equiv n^{(i)}$ with $i = 1, 2, \cdots, 22, X, Y, m, s$. It is useful to introduce chromosome pair

$$: C_{a_1}^{(i)}, C_{a_2}^{(i)} :$$

where the chromosome pair allele would run from 1 to $(n^{(i)} + 1)n^{(i)}/2$ with $i = 1, 2, \cdots, 22, X$, while Y chromosome and mitochondria do not need the pairing.

Integrating all, a female genotype $T_a^{(F)}$ and a male genotype $T_a^{(M)}$ are expressed in terms of chromosome pairs, mitochondria and a series of social genes having multiple alleles. We denote for a female genotype,

$$T_a^{(F)} = (C_{p_1}^{(1)}, C_{q_1}^{(1)} : \cdots : C_{p_{22}}^{(22)}, C_{q_{22}}^{(22)} : C_{p_X}^{(X)}, C_{q_X}^{(X)} : M_{p_m} : S_{p_s}).$$

Similarly, we denote for a male genotype,

$$T_a^{(M)} = (C_{p_1}^{(1)}, C_{q_1}^{(1)} : \cdots : C_{p_{22}}^{(22)}, C_{q_{22}}^{(22)} : C_{p_X}^{(X)}, C_{q_Y}^{(Y)} : M_{p_m} : S_{p_s}).$$

We find that the number of different genotypes is given by $[\prod_{i=1}^{22}\frac{1}{2}(1+n^{(i)})n^{(i)}]\frac{1}{2}(1+n^{(X)})n^{(X)}n^{(m)}n^{(s)}$ for female, and $[\prod_{i=1}^{22}\frac{1}{2}(1+n^{(i)})n^{(i)}]n^{(X)}n^{(Y)}n^{(m)}n^{(s)}$ for male. Note that, for several given genes, the number of distinguishable genotypes increases dramatically.

For a genotype $T_a^{(S)}$ with $S = F$ or M, we introduce four kinds of population ratios at the n-th generation: adult, birth, parent before mutation, and effective parent after mutation, which are denoted by $A_n(T_a^{(S)})$, $B_n(T_a^{(S)})$, $P_n(T_a^{(F)} \times T_b^{(M)})$, and $\widetilde{P}_n(T_a^{(F)} \times T_b^{(M)})$, respectively. Here, the population ratios denote the frequencies of specific genotypes or genotype pairs of parents. We normalize so that the sums of any population ratios are equal to 1 as shown in Table 1. We shall notice the relationships between these population ratios later.

The population evolution is governed by the four factors: (1) mating, (2) mutation, (3) reproduction, and (4) selection. We introduce some symbols used in the population evolution as follows in each step.

In mating, $\omega(T_a^{(F)} \to T_b^{(M)})$ denotes the probability that a genotype $T_a^{(F)}$ adult woman mates with a $T_b^{(M)}$ adult man, while $\omega(T_b^{(M)} \to T_a^{(F)})$ is the probability that a genotype $T_b^{(M)}$ adult man mates with a $T_a^{(F)}$ adult woman. This mating probability reflects social and cultural effects. For the random mating case, the probability $\omega(T_a^{(F)} \to T_b^{(M)})$ is simply $A_n(T_b^{(M)})$, and $\omega(T_b^{(M)} \to T_a^{(F)}) = A_n(T_a^{(F)})$. Notice that $\omega(T_a^{(F)} \to T_b^{(M)}) \neq \omega(T_b^{(M)} \to T_a^{(F)})$.

In mutation, the genotype mutation rates $\mu(T_a^{(S)} \to T_b^{(S)})$ are written in terms of the gene mutation rates $\mu(G_c^{(i,l)} \to G_d^{(i,l)})$ and the frequency of recombination due to chromosomal crossover. It is known that the frequency of recombination between two locations depends on their distance. Mutation rates between chromosomes are given by

$$\mu(C_a^{(i)} \to C_b^{(i)}) = \prod_{l=1}^{L} \mu(G_{a_l}^{(i,l)} \to G_{b_l}^{(i,l)}).$$

The mutation rates of mitochondria $\mu(M_a \to M_b)$ and the mutation rates of social gene string $\mu(S_a \to S_b)$ are given as the above similarly. Since each chromosome behaves independently, we find the mutation rate of a specific genotype $T_a^{(S)}$ with the sex index $S = F$ or M as

$$\mu(T_a^{(S)} \to T_b^{(S)}) = [\prod_{i=1}^{22} \eta^{(i)}]\eta^{(S)}\mu(M_{a_m} \to M_{b_m})\mu(S_{a_s} \to S_{b_s}),$$

where $\eta^{(i)} = \eta^{(i)}(C_v^{(i)}, C_w^{(i)} \to C_p^{(i)}, C_q^{(i)})$ is given by

$$\eta^{(i)} = \begin{cases} \mu(C_v^{(i)} \to C_p^{(i)})\mu(C_w^{(i)} \to C_p^{(i)}) & \text{for } p = q \\ \mu(C_v^{(i)} \to C_p^{(i)})\mu(C_w^{(i)} \to C_q^{(i)}) + \mu(C_v^{(i)} \to C_q^{(i)})\mu(C_w^{(i)} \to C_p^{(i)}) & \text{for } p \neq q \end{cases}$$

Furthermore, $\eta^{(F)}(C_v^{(X)}, C_w^{(X)} \to C_p^{(X)}, C_q^{(X)})$ is the same as $\eta^{(i)}$, and

$$\eta^{(M)}(C_v^{(X)}, C_w^{(Y)} \to C_p^{(X)}, C_q^{(Y)}) = \mu(C_v^{(X)} \to C_p^{(X)})\mu(C_w^{(Y)} \to C_q^{(Y)}).$$

For the social genes, mutation rates are mainly determined by the society and will be different for each case. In consequence, all genotype mutation rates are written in terms of the gene mutation rates. After mutation, the effective parent population $\widetilde{P}_n(T_a^{(F)} \times T_b^{(M)})$ will make offsprings.

In reproduction, the reproduction coefficients $\xi(T_b^{(F)} \times T_c^{(M)} \to T_a^{(S)})$ are calculated with the assumption that randomly chosen half of the father's chromosomes and half of the mother's chromosomes are delivered to their baby, however only the mother's mitochondria becomes the baby's mitochondria. For the social genes, the rule of reproduction will be different on a case-by-case basis. Assuming equal preference for each genotype, the reproduction coefficients $\xi(T_b^{(F)} \times T_c^{(M)} \to T_a^{(S)})$ can be calculated. In fact, the reproduction coefficients are written as

$$\xi(T_a^{(F)} \times T_b^{(M)} \to T_c^{(S)}) = [\prod_{i=1}^{22} \zeta^{(i)}]\zeta^{(S)}\zeta^{(m)}\zeta^{(s)}.$$

Here, $\zeta^{(i)} = \zeta^{(i)}(C_v^{(i)}, C_w^{(i)} \times C_p^{(i)}, C_q^{(i)} \to C_s^{(i)}, C_t^{(i)})$ is determined by the following simple algorithm:

Start with $\zeta^{(i)} = 0$.

If $(s,t) = (\mathtt{min}(v,p), \mathtt{max}(v,p))$, then add $\frac{1}{4}$ to $\zeta^{(i)}$.

If $(s,t) = (\mathtt{min}(v,q), \mathtt{max}(v,q))$, then add $\frac{1}{4}$ to $\zeta^{(i)}$.

If $(s,t) = (\mathtt{min}(w,p), \mathtt{max}(w,p))$, then add $\frac{1}{4}$ to $\zeta^{(i)}$.

If $(s,t) = (\mathtt{min}(w,q), \mathtt{max}(w,q))$, then add $\frac{1}{4}$ to $\zeta^{(i)}$.

Hence, $\zeta^{(i)}$ is given by one of four values, 0, $\frac{1}{4}$, $\frac{1}{2}$, 1. Also, $\zeta^{(F)}(C_v^{(X)}, C_w^{(X)} \times C_p^{(X)}, C_q^{(Y)} \to C_s^{(X)}, C_t^{(X)})$ is similarly determined:

Start with $\zeta^{(F)} = 0$.

If $(s,t) = (\mathtt{min}(v,p), \mathtt{max}(v,p))$, then add $\frac{1}{2}$ to $\zeta^{(F)}$.

If $(s,t) = (\mathtt{min}(w,p), \mathtt{max}(w,p))$, then add $\frac{1}{2}$ to $\zeta^{(F)}$.

Furthermore, $\zeta^{(M)}(C_v^{(X)}, C_w^{(X)} \times C_p^{(X)}, C_q^{(Y)} \to C_s^{(X)}, C_t^{(Y)})$ is determined as follows:

Start with $\zeta^{(M)} = 0$.

If $(s,t) = (v,q)$, then add $\frac{1}{2}$ to $\zeta^{(M)}$.

If $(s,t) = (w,q)$, then add $\frac{1}{2}$ to $\zeta^{(M)}$.

For mitochondria, $\zeta^{(m)}(M_v \times M_p \to M_s)$ is determined as follows:

Start with $\zeta^{(m)} = 0$.

If $s = v$, then add 1 to $\zeta^{(m)}$.

Finally, the reproduction coefficients $\zeta^{(s)}$ for social genes will be determined by a case-by-case consideration.

Name	Symbol	Property
Adult population	$A_n(T_a^{(S)})$	$\sum_a A_n(T_a^{(S)}) = 1$
Birth population	$B_n(T_a^{(S)})$	$\sum_a B_n(T_a^{(S)}) = 1$
Parents population	$P_n(T_a^{(F)} \times T_b^{(M)})$	$\sum_{a,b} P_n(T_a^{(F)} \times T_b^{(M)}) = 1$
Effective parents population	$\widetilde{P}_n(T_a^{(F)} \times T_b^{(M)})$	$\sum_{a,b} \widetilde{P}_n(T_a^{(F)} \times T_b^{(M)}) = 1$
Mating probability	$\omega(T_a^{(F)} \to T_b^{(M)})$	$\sum_b \omega(T_a^{(F)} \to T_b^{(M)}) = 1$
Genotype mutation rate	$\mu(T_a^{(S)} \to T_b^{(S)})$	$\sum_b \mu(T_a^{(S)} \to T_b^{(S)}) = 1$
Reproduction coefficient	$\xi(T_a^{(F)} \times T_b^{(M)} \to T_c^{(S)})$	$\sum_c \xi(T_a^{(F)} \times T_b^{(M)} \to T_c^{(S)}) = 1$
Disadvantage factor	$\delta(T_a^{(S)})$	$0.0 \leq \delta(T_a^{(S)}) \leq 1.0$

Table 1. Symbols used in the paper. The index S in genotype represents female with $S = F$, and male with $S = M$.

In selection, since human beings with faulty genes have lower survival rate, we introduce disadvantage factor $\delta(T_a^{(S)})$ for each genotype, which is given by a value between 0 and 1. A larger value of disadvantage factor means less chance of survival. The value of 1 represents the complete extinction. The terminology of fitness can alternatively be used to replace the disadvantage factor.

2.2 Population equation

For given population ratios $A_n(T_a^{(S)})$ at the n-th generation, our prime concern is "what are the next generation population ratios?". To answer this question, we introduce the four main effects on population evolution: mating, mutation, reproduction, and selection. Based on these four events, using the parameters in relation to probability as explained in the previous subsection, we formulate automata equations for population evolution:

• Mating

$$P_n(T_a^{(F)} \times T_b^{(M)}) = A_n(T_a^{(F)})\omega(T_a^{(F)} \to T_b^{(M)}) = A_n(T_b^{(M)})\omega(T_b^{(M)} \to T_a^{(F)}), \tag{1}$$

• Mutation

$$\widetilde{P}_n(T_a^{(F)} \times T_b^{(M)}) = \sum_{c,d} P_n(T_c^{(F)} \times T_d^{(M)})\mu(T_c^{(F)} \to T_a^{(F)})\mu(T_d^{(M)} \to T_b^{(M)}), \tag{2}$$

• Reproduction

$$B_n(T_a^{(S)}) = \sum_{b,c} \widetilde{P}_n(T_b^{(F)} \times T_c^{(M)})\xi(T_b^{(F)} \times T_c^{(M)} \to T_a^{(S)}), \tag{3}$$

• Selection

$$A_{n+1}(T_a^{(S)}) = \frac{B_n(T_a^{(S)})\{1 - \delta(T_a^{(S)})\}}{1 - \sum_b B_n(T_b^{(S)})\delta(T_b^{(S)})}. \tag{4}$$

The first equation is similar to the detailed balance in Monte Carlo simulation. The second equation shows that new populations are written as the sum of mutations from old

populations. The birth populations are determined in the third equation. The fractional adult populations at the next generation after selection and normalization are given by the fourth equation. These automata equations enable us to calculate the evolution of the genotype frequencies.

For a given initial normalized set of adult populations, the automata equations will produce a fixed point of $A^*(T_a^{(S)})$ eventually. We note that the fixed point has a global stability, and is a function of mutation rates and disadvantage factors. We present the entire library for solving the population equation on the Internet (Chung, 2007). In fact, written in C# language, the single reusable library of Science.dll contains Science.Biology.PopulationGenetics, with which one can simulate all cases. It is open to the public, and runs on a personal computer with Windows operating system. Any number of loci and alleles, and any values of mutation rates and disadvantage factors are allowed simultaneously.

It is worth mentioning that these population equations are not universal. In fact, if we introduce age as a social gene, these equations should be modified because only certain aged adults can marry and reproduce offsprings.

2.3 Non-random mating

While it is difficult to obtain detailed information on the biological genes of a prospective marriage partner, it is easy to do so on the social genes. Thus, the mating involving social genes will be a non-random mating in general.

In the population equation for mating of Eq. (1) which is analogous to detailed balance in the Monte Carlo simulation, the sum of probabilities must be 1. In fact, we require

$$\sum_b \omega(T_a^{(F)} \to T_b^{(M)}) = \sum_a \omega(T_b^{(M)} \to T_a^{(F)}) = 1. \tag{5}$$

Introducing a so-called *mating factor* Γ_{ab} which should not be negative, we rewrite the parent population as

$$P_n(T_a^{(F)} \times T_b^{(M)}) = A_n(T_a^{(F)})\Gamma_{ab}A_n(T_b^{(M)}). \tag{6}$$

Here, Γ_{ab} are input parameters in this model. However, the condition of Eq. (5) assures that the elements of Γ_{ab} should satisfy

$$\sum_{a=1}^{n^{(F)}} A_n(T_a^{(F)})\Gamma_{ab} = 1 \;\text{ for }\; 1 \le b \le n^{(M)}, \tag{7}$$

$$\sum_{b=1}^{n^{(M)}} \Gamma_{ab}A_n(T_b^{(M)}) = 1 \;\text{ for }\; 1 \le a \le n^{(F)}, \tag{8}$$

$$\Gamma_{ab} \ge 0. \tag{9}$$

These restrictions on Γ_{ab} assume that all adults marry and reproduce offsprings. When some genotype adults have handicaps for marriage, it is reflected in the disadvantage factor in selection.

Since we obtain the same equation from Eqs. (7) and (8) as

$$\sum_{ab} A_n(T_a^{(F)})\Gamma_{ab}A_n(T_b^{(M)}) = 1 = \sum_a A_n(T_a^{(F)}) = \sum_b A_n(T_b^{(M)}), \tag{10}$$

the constraint equations of Eqs. (7) and (8) are not linearly independent. We note that the number of constraints is given by $n^{(M)} + n^{(F)} - 1$. Hence, the number of free input parameters is given by $n^{(F)}n^{(M)} - n^{(M)} - n^{(F)} + 1$.

Although there are many ways to assign free parameters, we present here four cases for the mating factors.

• Random mating

A trivial but important solution would be the random mating for which all of Γ_{ab} are given by 1.

• Selective mating

If only one specific genotype is preferred completely, say $T_1^{(F)}$ and $T_1^{(M)}$, we let the free parameters of mating factors all zero as

$$(\Gamma_{ab}) = \begin{pmatrix} \Gamma_{11} & \Gamma_{12} & \Gamma_{13} & \cdots & \Gamma_{1n^{(M)}} \\ \Gamma_{21} & 0 & 0 & & 0 \\ \Gamma_{31} & 0 & 0 & & 0 \\ \vdots & & & \ddots & \vdots \\ \Gamma_{n^{(F)}1} & 0 & 0 & \cdots & 0 \end{pmatrix}. \tag{11}$$

In order to satisfy the constraints, other $n^{(M)} + n^{(F)} - 1$ factors should be given by

$$(\Gamma_{ab}) = \begin{pmatrix} \frac{-1+A_n(T_1^{(F)})+A_n(T_1^{(M)})}{A_n(T_1^{(F)})A_n(T_1^{(M)})} & \frac{1}{A_n(T_1^{(F)})} & \frac{1}{A_n(T_1^{(F)})} & \cdots & \frac{1}{A_n(T_1^{(F)})} \\ \frac{1}{A_n(T_1^{(M)})} & 0 & 0 & & 0 \\ \frac{1}{A_n(T_1^{(M)})} & 0 & 0 & & 0 \\ \vdots & & & \ddots & \vdots \\ \frac{1}{A_n(T_1^{(M)})} & 0 & 0 & \cdots & 0 \end{pmatrix}. \tag{12}$$

We note that the mating factors depend on population ratios at each generation. It should be emphasized from Γ_{11} that the population of $A_n(T_1^{(F)}) + A_n(T_1^{(M)})$ must be greater than 1 at the initial stage, and remains greater than 1 until the population ratios arrive at the equilibrium in this non-random mating.

• Hierarchical mating

For the case of $n^{(F)} = n^{(M)}$, we can define the mating factors as

$$(\Gamma_{ab}) = \begin{pmatrix} \Gamma_{11} & 0 & 0 & \cdots & 0 \\ \Gamma_{21} & \Gamma_{22} & 0 & & 0 \\ 0 & \Gamma_{32} & \Gamma_{33} & & 0 \\ \vdots & & & \ddots & \vdots \\ 0 & 0 & 0 & \cdots & \Gamma_{n^{(F)}n^{(M)}} \end{pmatrix}. \tag{13}$$

Here all the free input parameters of the mating factors are given by zero. The $n^{(M)} + n^{(F)} - 1$ factors should be determined by the constraints. As a result, we can determine Γ_{ab} as

$$\Gamma_{11} = \frac{1}{A_n(T_1^{(M)})}, \tag{14}$$

$$\Gamma_{21} = \frac{1}{A_n(T_2^{(F)})}(1 - \frac{A_n(T_1^{(F)})}{A_n(T_1^{(M)})}), \tag{15}$$
$$\cdots ,$$

where we omit presenting other Γ_{ab}, which have similar expressions in terms of the genotype frequencies.

• General non-random mating

We consider a new and more general approach by introducing the method of the linear programming.

When non-random mating is involved, there are $n^{(F)} \cdot n^{(M)}$ unknown values of Γ_{ab}. Since the number of the unknowns is bigger than the number of the restriction equations of Eqs. (7) and (8), there is no unique way to determine the mating factors Γ_{ab}. However, if we add a theoretical restriction such as maximization or minimization of a specific population, a unique process becomes possible. We introduce an additional condition of maximizing Z, which is written in terms of the parent populations as

$$Z = \sum_{ab} \beta_{ab} P_n(T_a^{(F)} \times T_b^{(M)}), \tag{16}$$

where the parameters β_{ab} represent the tendency of mating. In the process of maximizing Z, a given positive (negative) value of β_{ab} will produce a bigger (smaller) value of $P_n(T_a^{(F)} \times T_b^{(M)})$, which corresponds to inbreeding (outbreeding) between $T_a^{(F)}$ type female and $T_b^{(M)}$ type male. This problem of maximizing the objective function Z with the constraints of Eqs. (7)-(9) is well known, and can be solved as a linear programming problem, for example by the simplex method (Press et al., 1992).

The nature of β_{ab} values can be understood if we use practical demographic data, for example, incomes or divorce rates for parent groups. For instance, for the society that wants to reduce the divorce rates, it is possible to find the mating factors Γ_{ab} for the minimal divorce rate. If β_{ab} values represent incomes, we find the mating factors for the maximum income of the society. In this paper, we consider only medical screening.

3. Hemophilia

For hemophilia, the locus of the relevant gene called F8 is on X chromosome, and the gene has two alleles: normal X and abnormal X'. For female, three genotypes exist: normal XX, carrier XX', and disease $X'X'$. For male, there are two genotypes: normal XY, and disease $X'Y$. In the model of hemophilia, it is worthwhile to present all input parameters explicitly. First of

all, for the random mating, all of mating factors are given by 1 as

$$\Gamma_{ab} = 1.$$

The mutation rates are given by

$$\mu(X \to X') = \alpha, \;\; \mu(X \to X) = 1 - \alpha,$$
$$\mu(X' \to X) = \beta, \;\; \mu(X' \to X') = 1 - \beta.$$

The reproduction coefficients are found as

$$\xi(XX \times XY \to XX) = 1, \;\; \xi(XX \times XY \to XX') = 0, \;\; \xi(XX \times XY \to X'X') = 0,$$
$$\xi(XX \times X'Y \to XX) = 0, \;\; \xi(XX \times X'Y \to XX') = 1, \;\; \xi(XX \times X'Y \to X'X') = 0,$$
$$\xi(XX' \times XY \to XX) = 0.5, \;\; \xi(XX' \times XY \to XX') = 0.5, \;\; \xi(XX' \times XY \to X'X') = 0,$$
$$\xi(XX' \times X'Y \to XX) = 0, \;\; \xi(XX' \times X'Y \to XX') = 0.5, \;\; \xi(XX' \times X'Y \to X'X') = 0.5,$$
$$\xi(X'X' \times XY \to XX) = 0, \;\; \xi(X'X' \times XY \to XX') = 1, \;\; \xi(X'X' \times XY \to X'X') = 0,$$
$$\xi(X'X' \times X'Y \to XX) = 0, \;\; \xi(X'X' \times X'Y \to XX') = 0, \;\; \xi(X'X' \times X'Y \to X'X') = 1,$$
$$\xi(XX \times XY \to XY) = 1, \;\; \xi(XX \times XY \to X'Y) = 0,$$
$$\xi(XX \times X'Y \to XY) = 1, \;\; \xi(XX \times X'Y \to X'Y) = 0,$$
$$\xi(XX' \times XY \to XY) = 0.5, \;\; \xi(XX' \times XY \to X'Y) = 0.5,$$
$$\xi(XX' \times X'Y \to XY) = 0.5, \;\; \xi(XX' \times X'Y \to X'Y) = 0.5,$$
$$\xi(X'X' \times XY \to XY) = 0, \;\; \xi(X'X' \times XY \to X'Y) = 1,$$
$$\xi(X'X' \times X'Y \to XY) = 0, \;\; \xi(X'X' \times X'Y \to X'Y) = 1.$$

In the United States, about 17,000 people have hemophilia. About one in 7,500 live male births has hemophilia and about one in 25,000,000 live female births has hemophilia. From the data, we find that almost all female babies with hemophilia are dead during the pregnancy. Thus, it is natural to assign the disadvantage factors as

$$\delta(XX) = \delta(XX') = \delta(XY) = 0, \; \delta(X'X') = 1, \; \delta(X'Y) = \delta.$$

Note that we take $\delta = 0$ if male patients are completely cured. In the next subsections, we study the effect of male patient treatment by changing δ. The value of δ reflects the social development and standards of the general health care of particular geographical region where the hemophilia population is living.

3.1 Random mating with $\delta = 1$

The most natural case of hemophilia would be random mating with fatal mortality. In this case, we let $\delta(X'Y) = \delta = 1$. We now focus on mutation rates $\mu(X \to X') = \alpha$ and $\mu(X' \to X) = \beta$.

In fact, we determine the mutation rate $\mu(X \to X')$ as about 3.3×10^{-5} using the demographic data of birth population, $XY : X'Y = 0.9999 : 0.0001$. The population equation at $\alpha = 3.3 \times 10^{-5}$ shows that the equilibrium adult population is calculated as

$$\begin{aligned} XX : XX' : X'X' &= 0.999868 : 0.000132 : 0, \\ XY : X'Y &= 1 : 0, \end{aligned} \tag{17}$$

where the value of 0.000132 was rather insensitive on the value of β. We found that this low sensitivity originates from the severe disadvantage factor in hemophilia. Although there is a report for existence of a gene self-repairing mechanism in the process of evolution (Avise, 1993), we assume that self-repairing is very rare. Throughout this section hereafter, we simply let $\beta = 0.0$ and $\alpha = 3.3 \times 10^{-5}$ for hemophilia.

It is shown that these equilibrium population ratio values can be easily achieved not only analytically but also numerically (Lee et al., 2001). Numerical simulations show that these values become stable after about 100 generations, having no dependence on the initial state.

3.2 Random mating with $\delta = 0.1$

We consider the case where male patients of hemophilia can be treated so that some of them could lead normal lives, although a genetic defect remains intact. However, since female baby patients are dead during the pregnancy, it is assumed that there is still no cure for female patients as it stands at present. In fact, when the disadvantage factors are given by $\delta(XX) = \delta(XX') = \delta(XY) = 0$, $\delta(X'Y) = 0.1$, and $\delta(X'X') = 1$ with the same mutation rates as the above, we find the equilibrium population:

$$\begin{aligned} XX : XX' : X'X' &= 0.998121 : 0.001879 : 0, \\ XY : X'Y &= 0.999125 : 0.000875, \end{aligned} \tag{18}$$

in the random mating case where all $\Gamma_{ab} = 1$. These numbers will be used as references to study the effect of the non-random mating below.

Recently an interesting article (Stonebraker et al., 2010) on hemophilia prevalence in different countries was published. The prevalence (per 100,000 males) for high income countries was 12.8 ± 6.0 (mean $\pm$ SD) whereas it was 6.6 ± 4.8 for the rest of the world. Within a country, there was a strong trend of increasing prevalence over time: the prevalence for Canada ranged from 10.2 in 1989 to 14.2 in 2008 and for the United Kingdom it ranged from 9.3 in 1974 to 21.6 in 2006. The data are consistent with the fact that the cure results in increasing hemophilia prevalence.

3.3 Non-random mating with $\delta = 0.1$ in minimizing $P_n(XX' \times X'Y)$

Since rapid advances in molecular genetics have highlighted the potential use of genetic testing to screen for adult-onset chronic diseases (Burke et al., 2001), medical screening becomes more plausible.

We consider an artificial circumstance, where society-wide medical screening is available to control the mating factors. For example, we consider the case of hemophilia with a medical screening. The goal in this consideration is to find the equilibrium populations in that society. We assume that the medical screening helps male patients avoid marrying disease carrier

women. This restriction lead us to choose the objective function as

$$Z = -P_n(XX' \times X'Y),$$

with which we expect a minimal value of $P_n(XX' \times X'Y)$ for maximizing Z. In consequence, with the previous disadvantage factors and mutation rates, the population equations give the equilibrium as

$$\begin{aligned} XX : XX' : X'X' &= 0.998089 : 0.001911 : 0, \\ XY : X'Y &= 0.999110 : 0.000890. \end{aligned} \tag{19}$$

The corresponding objective function Z is given by simply 0 as expected. We find the different numbers of the male patients and the female carriers from those of the random mating in Eq. (18).

3.4 Non-random mating with $\delta = 0.1$ in maximizing $\mathbf{P}_n(\mathbf{XX'}\times\mathbf{X'Y})$

It is instructive to compare the above result with that of the opposite situation where the objective function is given by

$$Z = P_n(XX' \times X'Y)$$

to maximize $P_n(XX' \times X'Y)$. For the same disadvantage factors and mutation rates as the above, the population equation gives the equilibrium as

$$\begin{aligned} XX : XX' : X'X' &= 0.999868 : 0.000132 : 0, \\ XY : X'Y &= 0.999911 : 0.000089. \end{aligned} \tag{20}$$

The corresponding objective function Z at equilibrium is given by 8.90937×10^{-5}, which means that all male patients marry with female carriers because $X'Y$ is given by 0.000089 as shown in the above.

We find that the population ratios of Eq. (18) in random mating are between two extremal cases of Eqs. (19) and (20), which correspond to outbreeding and inbreeding of female carriers and male patients, respectively.

3.5 Non-random mating in association of a social gene

We now consider the effect of the social inheritance on the evolution of the biological genes in the case of hemophilia. We consider a two-gene system, where one of the relevant genes is hemophilia on X chromosome, and the other is a social gene. For simplicity, we assume that the social gene has two allele: Rich(R) and Poor(P). In this model, there are six female genotypes and four male genotypes:

$$\begin{aligned} T_1^{(F)} &= XX : R, \quad T_2^{(F)} = XX : P, \\ T_3^{(F)} &= X'X : R, \quad T_4^{(F)} = X'X : P, \\ T_5^{(F)} &= X'X' : R, \quad T_6^{(F)} = X'X' : P, \\ T_1^{(M)} &= XY : R, \quad T_2^{(M)} = XY : P, \\ T_3^{(M)} &= X'Y : R, \quad T_4^{(M)} = X'Y : P. \end{aligned} \tag{21}$$

For the biological gene, we use the same mutation rates $\mu(X \to X')$, $\mu(X' \to X)$ and the same reproduction rates $\xi^{(b)}$ as before.
For the social gene, we let the mutation rates be

$$\mu(R \to P) = 0.2 \text{ and } \mu(P \to R) = 0.1 \tag{22}$$

as a sample example. Also, we assign the reproduction rates $\xi^{(s)}$ with which the whole reproduction rates ξ in the population equations are written as $\xi = \xi^{(b)}\xi^{(s)}$:

$$\begin{aligned}
\xi^{(s)}(R \times R \to R) = 1,\ \xi^{(s)}(R \times R \to P) = 0,\\
\xi^{(s)}(R \times P \to R) = 1,\ \xi^{(s)}(R \times P \to P) = 0,\\
\xi^{(s)}(P \times R \to R) = 1,\ \xi^{(s)}(P \times R \to P) = 0,\\
\xi^{(s)}(P \times P \to R) = 0,\ \xi^{(s)}(P \times P \to P) = 1.
\end{aligned} \tag{23}$$

We further assign the disadvantage factors as

$$\begin{aligned}
\delta(T_1^{(F)}) = 0,\ \delta(T_2^{(F)}) = 0,\\
\delta(T_3^{(F)}) = 0,\ \delta(T_4^{(F)}) = 0,\\
\delta(T_5^{(F)}) = 1,\ \delta(T_6^{(F)}) = 1,\\
\delta(T_1^{(M)}) = 0,\ \delta(T_2^{(M)}) = 0,\\
\delta(T_3^{(M)}) = 0,\ \delta(T_4^{(M)}) = 0.1.
\end{aligned} \tag{24}$$

These factors imply that hemophilia is still fatal for female patients, while the rich social gene can make male patients lead normal lives.
In order to analyze equilibrium population resulted from inbreeding between the normal and rich genotypes, we set the objective function as

$$Z = P_n(T_1^{(F)} \times T_1^{(M)}).$$

With all the given parameters as the above with the inbreeding, we find the equilibrium population ratios as

$$\begin{aligned}
&T_1^{(F)} : T_2^{(F)} : T_3^{(F)} : T_4^{(F)} : T_5^{(F)} : T_6^{(F)}\\
&\quad = 0.833195 : 0.154462 : 0.009700 : 0.002643 : 0 : 0,\\
&T_1^{(M)} : T_2^{(M)} : T_3^{(M)} : T_4^{(M)}\\
&\quad = 0.837755 : 0.156138 : 0.005223 : 0.000884.
\end{aligned} \tag{25}$$

We clearly observe that the existence of social gene drastically influences the inheritance of the biological genes. We believe that this influence is induced by the disadvantage factor of the genotype, $T_4^{(M)}$.
In order to examine the role of the disadvantage factor in the evolution mechanism, we have carried out a calculation by changing only $\delta(T_4^{(M)})$ from 0.1 to 1. The resulting population

ratios are given by

$$\begin{aligned} &T_1^{(F)} : T_2^{(F)} : T_3^{(F)} : T_4^{(F)} : T_5^{(F)} : T_6^{(F)} \\ &\quad = 0.826752 : 0.171908 : 0.001127 : 0.000213 : 0 : 0, \\ &T_1^{(M)} : T_2^{(M)} : T_3^{(M)} : T_4^{(M)} \\ &\quad = 0.827356 : 0.172040 : 0.000604 : 0. \end{aligned} \tag{26}$$

Comparing with Eq. (25), we clearly observe that the change of the disadvantage factor has a significant influence on the hemophiliac biological evolution. We also note that the ratio of rich to poor is higher in the diseased than in the healthy, clearly indicating the social gene effect of richness. Thus, we note again that existence of a particular social gene can have significant effect on the evolution process.

We note that a drawback of our approach is in the large number of tunable parameters. While mutation rates and recombination rates for biological genes may be adjusted by the coalescent method, it is hard to find an empirical basis for social genes. The social gene of last name probably gains some empirical support. However, if no support is provided, it is reasonable to perform sensitivity analysis by scanning around chosen parameters.

There are many genetic diseases other than hemophilia in the real world. As an example, the same approach may be applied to the case of congenital hypothyroidism (Calaciura et al., 2002). Expansion of the present scheme to other cases including more diverse social genes remains as a future study.

4. Conclusion

We have presented a theoretical scheme and a simulation program to study population genetics in a realistic complex situation. The result shows that the multiplicity of the gene loci greatly affect the demographic distribution of fractional population ratios. We suggest that more detailed demographic data including gene mutation (Porter, 1968; Strachan, 1996) and fitness is desirable to elaborate the theory further.

Treating social status as an inheritance trait, we introduce the concept of the social gene. Treating the social genes on equal footing with the biological genes, we build a unified framework to find the population evolution (Cavalli-Sforza & Bodmer, 1996) in the biological and the social inheritance. The nature of the social inheritance inevitably introduces the concept of non-random mating. This framework is used to investigate the detailed cases of hemophilia.

For hemophilia, we have presented a theoretical scheme to determine the mating factors uniquely in the non-random mating process by introducing the objective function concept. Finally, we have considered the effect of the social gene with two alleles, Rich and Poor on the biological gene of hemophilia. The result shows that the introduction of a social gene or social inheritances change the population evolution of the biological gene. We note that the social gene concept introduced here is different from polyphenism, for which multiple phenotypes can arise from a single genotype as a result of differing environment conditions. The reason for the difference is that the social gene is inherited with the biological gene, whereas the environment is not.

The current study does not include any dynamic change of mutation factors, which are expected especially in the social gene inheritance. The collective and the dynamic behavior are subjects of future studies.

5. References

Alpern, S. & Reyniers, D. (2005). Strategic mating with common preferences. *Journal of Theoretical Biology*, 237 : 337-354.

Aoki, K. (2001). Theoretical and empirical aspects of gene-culture coevolution. *Theoretical Population Biology*, 59 : 253-261.

Avise, J.C. (1993). The evolutionary biology of aging, sexual reproduction, and DNA repair. *Evolution*, 47 : 1293-1301.

Bamshad, M.J. et al. (1998). Female gene flow stratifies hindu castes. *Nature*, 395 : 651-652.

Burke, W.; Coughlin, S.S.; Lee, N.C.; Weed, D.L. & Khoury, M.J. (2001). Application of population screening principles to genetic screening for adult-onset conditions. *Genetic Testing*, 5 : 201-211.

Calaciura, F. et al. (2002). Genetics of specific phenotypes of congenital hypothyroidism: a population-based approach. *Thyroid*, 12 : 945-951.

Cavalli-Sforza, L.L. & Bodmer, W.F. (1971). *The Genetics of Human Populations*, W. H. Freeman and Company, San Francisco.

Cavalli-Sforza, L.L. & Feldman, M.W. (1981). *Cultural Transmission and Evolution: A quantitative approach*, Princeton University Press, New Jersey.

Charlesworth, B. (1994). *Evolution in age-structured populations second edition*, Cambridge University Press, Cambridge.

Chung, M.-H.; Lee, S.P.; Kim, C.K. & Nahm, K. (1997). Fractional populations of blood groups. *Physical Review E*, 56 : 865-869.

Chung, M.H.; Kim, C.K. & Nahm, K. (2003). Fractional populations in multiple gene inheritance. *Bioinformatics*, 19 : 256-260.

Chung, M.H. (2007). http://www.sciencecode.com/populationgenetics.htm.

Chung, M.H.; Kim, C.K. (2010). Non-random mating involving inheritance of social status. *Journal of Computational Biology*, 17 : 745-754.

Fu, Y.X. & Li, W.H. (1999). Minireview: coalescing into the 21st century: an overview and prospects of coalescent theory. *Theoretical Population Biology*, 56 : 1-10.

Haldane, J.B.S. (1935). The rate of spontaneous mutation of a human gene. *Journal of Genetics*, 31 : 317-326.

Hampe, J.; Wienker, T.; Schreiber, S. & Nürnberg, P. (1998). POPSIM: a general population simulation program. *Bioinformatics*, 14 : 458-464.

Hausken, K. & Hirshleifer, J. (2001). The truthful signalling hypothesis: an explicit general equilibrium model. *Journal of Theoretical Biology*, 228 : 497-511.

Hedrick, P.W. (1985). *Genetics of Populations*, Jones And Bartlett Publishers, Boston.

Hudson, R.R. (1991). *Oxford Surveys in Evolutionary Biology Vol. 7*, Cambridge University Press, Cambridge, pp. 1-44.

Lander, E.S. et al. (2001). Initial sequencing and analysis of the human genome. *Nature*, 409 : 860-921.

Lee, S.P.; Chung, M.-H.; Kim, C.K. & Nahm, K. (2001). Fractional populations in sex-linked inheritance. *Physica A*, 291 : 533-541.

Li, C.C. (1976). *First Course in Population Genetics*, Boxwood, Pacific Grove.
Mekjian, D.A.Z. (1991). Cluster distributions in physics and genetic diversity. *Physical Review A*, 44 : 8361-8374.
Möhle, M. & Sagitov, S. (2003). Coalescent patterns in exchangeable diploid population models. *Journal of Mathematical Biology*, 47 : 337-352.
Nagylaki, T.; Hofbauer, J. & Brunovský, P. (1999). Convergence of multilocus systems under weak epistasis or weak selection. *Journal of Mathematical Biology*, 38 : 103-133.
National Hemophilia Foundation. (1998). http://www.hemophilia.org.
Perelson, A.S. & Weisbuch, G. (1997). Immunology for physicists. *Reviews of Modern Physics*, 69 : 1219-1267.
Piccolboni, A. & Gusfield, D. (2003). On the Complexity of Fundamental Computational Problems in Pedigree Analysis. *Journal of Computatinal Biology*, 10 : 763-774.
Porter, I.H. (1968). *Heredity and Disease*, McGraw-Hill, New York.
Press, W.H.; Teukolsky, S.A.; Vetterling, W.T. & Flannery, B.P. (1992). *Numerical recipes in C second edition*, Cambridge University Press, Cambridge, pp. 430-444.
Quardokus, E. (2000). Modeling population genetics. *Science*, 288 : 458-459.
Radcliffe, J. & Rass, L. (1999). Strategic and genetic models of evolution. *Mathematical Biosciences*, 156 : 291-307.
Rosenberg, N.A. & Nordborg, M.N. (2002). Genealogical trees, coalescent theory and the analysis of genetic polymorphisms. *Nature Reviews Genetics*, 3 : 380-390.
Santafe, G.; Lozano, J.A. & Larranaga, P. (2008). Inference of Population Structure Using Genetic Markers and a Bayesian Model Averaging Approach for Clustering. *Journal of Computational Biology*, 15 : 207-220.
Stonebraker, J.S.; Bolton-Maggs, P.H.B.; Michael Soucie, J.; Walker, I. & Brooker, M. (2010). A study of variations in the reported haemophilia A prevalence around the world. *Haemophilia*, 16 : 20-32.
Strachan, T. & Read, A.P. (1996). *Human Molecular Genetics*, Bios Scientific Publishers, Oxford.
Thomson, R.; Pritchard, J.K.; Shen, P.; Oefner, P.J. & Feldman, M.W. (2000). *Proceedings of the National Academy of Sciences*, 97 : 7360-7365.
Venter, J.C. et al. (2001). The sequence of the human genome. *Science*, 291 : 1304-1351.

5

Hemophilia Inhibitors Prevalence, Causes and Diagnosis

Tarek M. Owaidah
King Faisal Specialist Hospital and RC
Saudi Arabia

1. Introduction

Hemophilia is a bleeding disorder that results from genetic alteration in production of coagulation factors that are important to maintain hemostasis. The commonest type is hemophilia A due to deficiency of factor VIII (FVIII), which is important zymogen co factor for clot formation. Hemophilia A is an X-linked disease that affects males at prevalence of 1:5000-10000. Hemophilia B is due to deficiency in factor (FIX) but less common with prevalence of 1:34,500 males. It is inherited also as X- linked. Although both disorders are rarely observed; they can be very serious (life threatening) and costly for families and countries. Treatment of hemophilia is based on replacement of the deficient factor. Two types of factor concentrates are available, plasma derived (pdFVIII/IX) and recombinant (rFVIII/IX) which are associated with variable incidence of inhibitor formation rates.The development of inhibitor is the most serious and challenging complication of hemophilia treatment with the enormous economic burden (1). FVIII inhibitors are immunoglobulin IgG (IgG1 and IgG4) antibodies that neutralize FVIII procoagulant activity in plasma. Inhibitors are usually classified according to their levels in plasma as a "high-titer" inhibitors, those with the highest activity >5 Bethesda Units (BU)/ml or a low-titer inhibitor type. In hemophilia A aproximately 60-70% of inhibitors are high titer inhibitors, and the remainder are low titer. Some patients develop transient inhibitors (usually low titer inhibitors that never exceed a titer of 5 BU/ml and disappear spontaneously with time (2). The development of inhibitors is associated with changes in the clinical picture with major effect on bleeding control, arthropathy status and overall quality of life. Patients with mild or moderate hemophilia may change to severe clinical behavior because of increase in factor clearance. Patients with inhibitors are resistant to the replacement therapy and thereby their bleeding symptoms become difficult to control and require either large doses of FVIII/IX or alternative hemostatic therapy with bypassing agents.
During almost 50 years many studies have addressed different aspects of inhibitors issue from risk factors to diagnosis and management of patients who developed these antibodies.

2. Type of factor inhibitors

Coagulation factor inhibitors can be divided to neutralizing antibodies that result in inactivation of the factor and non-neutralizing (i.e. non-inhibitory) antibodies that target non-functional epitopes on FVIII. The non-neutralizing antibodies become clinically relevant if they result in accelerated clearance of the transfused clotting factor (3) . Both types can by classified as:

a. alloantibodies, those that develop in hemophiliacs exposed to exogenous FVIII or FIX. Most FVIII alloantibodies are directed against epitopes in the A2 and A3-C1 domains of FVIII. This binding interferes with the assembly of the FVIII-FIX complex. Antibodies directed against C2 domain affect the binding of FVIII to phospholipid and von Willebrand factor (vWF) and interfere with cleavage of FVIII by thrombin and FXa. In vitro the inactivation of factor VIII is time, temperature and pH dependent (4). Alloantibodies have type 1 reaction kinetics, which means that all FVIII added to haemophilia plasma is inhibited lineary.
b. autoantibodies, those that suddenly appear in persons with normal F8 gene and previously normal plasma levels of FVIII, causing so called "acquired hemophilia". These inhibitors occur predominantly in the elderly patients, patients with autoimmune, inflammatory process and lymphoprolipherative disorders, and rarely in association with pregnancy (5,6) and result in serious bleeding manifestation with a high morbidity and mortality of 6%-20%. Currently 70%-80% of cases of acquired hemophilia are successfully treated with immunosuppressive therapy (7,8). In vitro FVIII autoantibodies present type 2 reactive kinetics with exponential decrease of FVIII, while even at a high titre of inhibitor some residual activity of factor may be detectable. (4)

Occasionally, alloantibodies may be mistaken for autoantibodies. This occurs when an individual with a clinically silent mutation in FVIII (for example, a B-domain mutation) is exposed to wild-type FVIII. (4)

3. Prevalence of inhibitor formation

The overall prevalence of inhibitors is up to 30% in patients with hemophilia A and up to 5% in those with hemophilia B (9). Inhibitors are reported rarely in other coagulation factor deficiencies. Data on 294 individuals with deficiencies of FII, FV, FVII, FX, FXIII from North American Rare Bleeding Disorder Registry reported only 3% of patients with FV and FXIII deficiency who developed inhibitors following infusion of FFP and FXIII concentrate (10).

Risk factors for inhibitor development can be patient related (genetic, ethnicity or immune system), treatment related (type of product, exposure to FVIII/IX in terms of the age at the first treatment, treatment duration and intensity) or diagnostics related (type and sensitivity of test detecting the inhibitor, frequency of inhibitor testing). There are differences between the prevalence and incidence of factor VIII/IX inhibitors. Earlier studies reported consistently the incidence of inhibitor in the range of 25%-32%, although the prevalence eventually fell to approximately 12% as some antibodies disappeared over time (3). Some reports used both terminologies interchangeably which could be explained by difficulty to investigate inhibitor incidence due to the need for high patient number in a relatively uncommon disease. However, early studies were often undertaken on selected patients populations, using different assays for inhibitor detection and being mostly one-off studies on the proportion of inhibitors in particular patient population at a given time (11).

In several cohort studies an incidence rate of new inhibitors (number of new cases/ population at risk x the time at which new cases were ascertained) was determined in the absence of new product exposure with different incidence results. As an example, Kempton et al (2006) reported incidence rate of factor VIII inhibitors of 2.14 per 1000 person-years (12).

4. Factors affecting development of inhibitors

Several risk factors for inhibitor formation have been hypothesized. Identification of these factors may help to predict inhibitor develoment and to choose the treatment approach minimising the potential risk in particular patient. The risk of developing inhibitors varies throughout the lifetime of a patient with haemophilia, with historical evidence suggesting that most of inhibitors develop during childhood before reaching the age of 12 years (13). The risk factors interact with each other and can be classified as "non-modifiable" and environmental, or so called "modifiable" risk factors.(14)

a) Non modifiable risk factors.

These patient related factors that may enhance the risk of inhibitor development include a high-risk hemophilia genotype, co-stimulatory genotype–immunogenotype interactions, ethnicity and positive family history [15,16,17].

Mutations in FVIII are major risk factors of inhibitor development predominantly in patients with severe form of disease (18). Several gene defects that increase the risk of factor VIII/IX inhibitors have been identified. Some mutations (so called null mutations) result in severe molecular defects with complete failure of FVIII or FIX proteins synthesis. High risk mutations include multi-domain mutations, large deletions/insertions and nonsense mutations which represent approximately 8% of all mutations in severe haemophilia A, as well as the intron-22 inversion with a prevalence of around 50%. The inhibitor formation in patients with high risk mutations ranges between 25% (intron 22 inv) and 60%-80% (multidomain mutations and large deletions) (17,18,).

Small deletions, missense and splice site mutations result in partial absence of FVIII protein and their prevalence in severe hemophilia is approximately 35% (19). Also in haemophilia B the genotype is a strong determinant of inhibitor risk; patients with gene deletions or rearrangements are at high risk of inhibitor formation. These mutations are present in approximately 50% of inhibitor patients, while the frameshift, premature stop, or splice-site mutations are present in approximately 20% of patients with inhibitor of FIX. The missense mutations, which constitute the majority of genotypes in haemophilia B are at very low risk of inhibitor formation (3,20). The prevalence of inhibitors in patients with haemophilia B and null mutations ranges from 6–60% (17).

The discordance of inhibitor development and the type of mutation has been observed in patients with the same mutation of the F8 or F9 gene, including the siblings, suggesting the involvement of other genetic and environmental risk factors that may prevent or facilitate inhibitor formation (21).

Polymorphisms of the immune response genes, including the genes encoding the major histocompatibility complex (MHC) class II system, tumor necrosis factor-α(TNF-α), interleukin-10 (IL-10) and cytotoxic T-lymphocyte antigen-4 (CTLA-4), have been suggested to be the factors contributing to the risk of inhibitor (22,23,24,25). Some specific types of (HLA) genes may also be implicated in increasing the risk of inhibitor development (26).

Ethnicity was also shown to play a role in development of inhibitors. African-Americans and Latinos with haemophilia A have higher inhibitor risk than Caucasians with prevalence of inhibitors in Black patients with hemophilia A twice of white patients (27,28). The estimated incidence of new inhibitors in Finnish patients was 10.3 per thousand patient years (29). In another study on inhibitors in Japanese populations the prevalence was as high as 29.7% (30). In a close population the prevalence of inhibitors in Chinese was as low

as 3.9% in hemophilia A and 4.3% in severe cases (31). It was interesting to find a high frequency (39.2%) of very low titer of inhibitors (<1 BU mL 1) in Chinese population which was seen also in a cohort of Saudi patients (32). There are few reports about the prevalence of these inhibitors in other ethnicity like Arabs. Recent epidemiological survey of the presence of inhibitors in known cases of Saudi hemophilia A and B showed a prevalence of inhibitors of 22% and 0%, respectively (32).

b) Modifiable risk factors

These include environmental influences that are implicated in increasing the risk of inhibitor formation. Identifying the environmental risk factors implicated in increasing the probability of inhibitor development permit anticipation of disease progression and allow the potential to intervene, and thereby modify patient treatment and improve the outcomes.

Environmental factors include, age at start of prophylaxis, type of replacement therapy product and intensity of treatment (28,33). Data from several studies have supported the idea that first replacement therapy at an early age may increase the risk of inhibitor formation (34, 35, 36). These studies showed that most inhibitors develop in children with severe hemophilia at the age of 1-2 years after 9-12 treatments. More recent large studies like the CANAL study (37) and Chalmers study (38) investigated the relationship between inhibitor development and treatment characteristics in previously untreated patients (PUPs) with severe haemophilia A and confirmed that an early age of first exposure to FVIII was associated with an increased risk of inhibitor development, however, further analysis showed that after adjustment for intensity of treatment and genetic factors, this association disappeared (37,38).

Gouw et al (2007) reported a cumulative incidence of clinically relevant inhibitor of 41% in patients starting therapy before the age of 1 month, 30% in patients starting therapy between 1 and 6 months of age, 23% in patients starting therapy between 6 and 12 months of age, 20% in patients starting therapy between 12 and 18 months, and 18% in those starting therapy beyond 18 months of age, respectively. However, the same findings of disappearance of the association between inhibiors and the age of the first treatment were observed after the adjustment for other confounding factors (39).

5. The effect of type of factor concentrates on inhibitor formation

The influence of the type of FVIII concentrate in PUPs with severe hemophilia A is highly controversial due to presence of different types of these products and methodological differences between studies which rendered comparisons inconclusive (14,28 40, 41). Purified factor VIII products were developed in the 1960s and become available as concentrates for reconstitution in the 1970's. Most of the early studies addressed the role of pd-FVIII in the development of inhibitor with a cumulative incidence of inhibitors ranging from 20.3% to 33.0% in PUPs exposed to different brands of low or intermediate purity pdFVIII concentrates (31 42, 43, 44). Further studies evaluating the inhibitor formation after pdFVIII products focused on the purity of factor VIII products as a potential risk factor. Purity of FVIII concentrates is defined as the biologic activity of FVIII:C (IU) per mg of total protein. The studies of patients treated with a single plasma-derived high purity antihemophilic factor concentrate containing vWF (Alphanate®, Humate-P®, Koate®-HP) showed the incidence of inhibitors in the range from 0% to 12.4% (45,46 47, 48 ,49). Most of

the current high purity pd-FVIII products carry almost 0% risk of inhibitor formation (50, 51). There is data supporting the protective effect of vWF, a carrier protein of FVIII which is present in a large amount in most pd-FVIII products but not in rFVIII, on inhibitor formation by reducing the immunogenicity of FVIII through preventing its entry into professional antigen presenting cells (52).

Recombinant factor VIII products became available in the early 1990's after the discovery of F8 gene in 1984. The cumulative risk of inhibitors in patients treated with first generation, single rFVIII product was reported to range from 32.0% to 38.7% (53,54,55). More recent studies have shown that in patients treated with the second generation rFVIII products the incidence of inhibitors ranged from 16.7 to 32% (28,56). Choosing a product for factor replacement is crucial, which sometimes creates pressure on the treating physician. The safety of the blood product is weighted against other factors like availability and cost of products and the risk of inhibitor formation. Goudemand et al (2006) demonstrated that high-purity pdFVIII concentrates containing von Willebrand factor have lower risk of inhibitor development compared with rFVIII. Adjusted relative risk for inhibitor with rFVIII was 2.4 for all inhibitors and 2.6 for high titre inhibitors when compared with pdFVIII (28). In a systematic review of 24 international studies published between 1970-2009, Iorio et al (2010) reported a pooled inhibitor incidence rate of 14.3% for pdFVIII and 27.4% for rFVIII, with the high titre inhibitor incidence of 9.3% for pdFVIII and 17.4% for rFVIII (57). In a more recent meta-analysis by Franchini et al (2011) evaluating the data from a total of 800 patients enrolled in 25 prospective studies published between 1990 and 2007, the incidence of inhibitors did not differ significantly in recipients of plasma derived and recombinant FVIII concentrates (58) . The authors concluded that type of product does not seem to influence the inhibitor development in PUPs with severe hemophilia A (58). Poon MC et al (2002) showed the same incidence of inhibitor formation in hemophilia B patients treated with rFIX and pdFIX concentrates (59).

The major limitation of all these reviews is that they compare different plasma derived and recombinant products used in different time periods with different approaches to treatment but also to the monitoring of inhibitors.

The lack of unbiased information on this issue was the driving force behind the SIPPET study (Study on Inhibitors in Plasma-Product Exposed Toddlers). This ongoing international, prospective, controlled (open-label) and randomized clinical trial is aimed to compare the immunogenicity of plasma-derived vWF/FVIII products with recombinant FVIII concentrates, by determining the frequency of inhibitor development in PUPs and minimally treated patients (MTPs) (60,61).

Intensity of treatment has been implicated as a factor responsible for increasing the risk for inhibitor development (62). In CANAL study it was shown that adjustment for intensity of treatment overcomes the effect of age on the development of inhibitor (39). Gouw et al (2007) showed in a multicentre cohort study that intensive treatment periods (peak treatment moments and surgical procedures) increase the risk of inhibitor formation (63). Furthermore, reduced interval between exposure days (EDs) was significantly associated with increased risk of inhibitor development with adjusted relative risk of 1.0 for >100 days between EDs vs. 2.5 and 2.7 for 10–100 days and <10 days respectively (63). The highest risk of developing inhibitors is observed within the first 50 exposures to FVIII, while the risk is substantially reduced after 200 treatment days (14).

Lack of standardization of the category "previously treated patients" (PTP) has led to many different reports on the inhibitors formation in this patients population (64). Nevertheless,, current FDA approach recommends to use the incidence of inhibitor formation in PTPs as the main criteria in the safety analysis of new FVIII products.
The International Society of Thrombosis and Haemostasis Scientific Subcommittee (ISTH) defines PTPs as patients with >150 lifetime exposure days (65), but this definition has not been used strictly in the studies evaluating the incidence of inhibitor formation after exposure to factor concentrates in previously treated patients. In these studies different definitions of PTPs were used with a number of ED ranging from a single exposure to >250 ED (66,67).
Some virus inactivation steps introduced in the early 1990´s with the aim to improve the safety of FVIII concentrates increased the immunogenicity of products and resulted in inhibitor formation in PTPs. Peerlinck et al (1993) and Rosendaal et al (1997) reported sudden increase of inhibitor formation in PTPs after the treatment with pasteurized intermediate purity FVIII concentrate. Incidence of inhibitors was 31 and 20.1 per 1000 person years in Belgium and the Netherlands, respectively (68,69).
Changes in the use of products created a new research area focused on inhibitors in patients who have switched one product for another FVIII concentrate. In two Canadian surveillance studies that evaluated inhibitor formation in PTPs following the switch of pdFVIII for rFVIII, the inhibitor incidence was similar to that seen in Canada prior to the introduction of recombinant products (70,71). This was also confirmed by more recent studies. Gouw et al (2007) in the CANAL study showed that switching between factor VIII products did not increase the risk for inhibitors (39). Some of postmarketing studies evaluated the switch for the newer generation concentrates of the same class products. Vidovic et al (2009) evaluated patients switching from Kogenate® (Bayer) for Kogenate FS® (Bayer) and did not find any inhibitors in the 185 subjects monitored for 2 years (72).

6. Diagnosis of inhibitors

The tests for detection of FVIII antibodies, based on mixing the patient´s and normal plasma underwent several modifications to improve their sensitivity. The first assay to determine the potency of inhibitor was described in 1959. This assay was quite accurate but required considerable technical skill and was beyond the capability of most clinical laboratories. Later investigators with an interest in haemophilia met in Bethesda and established a method for measurement of FVIII inhibitors (73). The assay was named Bethesda assay and was based on the ability of antibody-containing plasma to inactivate the FVIII of pooled normal plasma. This assay has become a standard test to measure clinically significant FVIII inhibitors. However, it has some limitations. The assay may not detect weak and non-neutralizing antibodies. Verbruggen B et al (1995) descried a modified Bethesda assay, the Nijmegen low titre inhibitor assay (74). Two modifications of the original method were adopted to overcome the poor specificity and imperfection of Bethesda assay, especially at the low levels of inhibitor: 1) buffering of normal plasma used in the assay and control mixture, with 0.1 M imidazole to pH 7.4 prevents the pH change occurring during the 2 hours incubation, and 2) replacing the imidazole buffer in the control mixture by immunodepleted FVIII deficient plasma increases the precision of the method . The Factor VIII/IX Subcommittee of the ISTH has endorsed the recommendation that the Nijmegen-modified Bethesda assay should be adopted to quantify FVIII inhibitors (75). Several

problems with FVIII inhibitor assay have not yet been resolved including: 1) the high interlaboratory variability in the quantification of FVIII inhibitors when the reference antibody standard is unavailable; 2) inability to identify the proportion of 'non-inhibitory' FVIII inhibitors leading to accelerated clearance of FVIII in vivo; and 3) the effect of the type of FVIII-deficient plasma on FVIII inhibitor detection. Verbruggen B et al (2001) showed that chemically depleted factor VIII deficient plasma can give falsely elevated titres when used in combination with other types of deficient plasmas as a substrate plasma in the factor VIII:C assay due to the presence of activated factor V in the preparation (76).
Several new tests have been developed recently to overcome the limitations of the Bethesda assay. ELISA-based assay for detection of FVIII-specific IgG was validated and found to have a strong correlation with Bethesda method in detecting immune response to FVIII. The ELISA provides rapid screening that could be available well in advance of inhibitor confirmation by the Bethesda assay (77,78). Recently developed a new fluorescence-based immunoassay (FLI) was found to be much more sensitive for detecting especially low titre inhibitors (79).

7. References

[1] Gringeri A, Mantovani LG, Scalone L, Mannucci PM. for the COCIS Study Group. Cost of care and quality of life for patients with hemophilia complicated by inhibitors: the COCIS Study Group Blood 2003; 102, 7:2358-63.
[2] White GC 2nd, Rosendaal F, Aledort LM, Lusher JM, Rothschild C, Ingerslev J; Factor VIII and Factor IX Subcommittee. Definitions in hemophilia. Recommendation of the scientific subcommittee on factor V III and factor IX of the scientific and standardization committee of the International Society on Thrombosis and Haemostasis. ThrombHaemost 2001; 85(3):560.
[3] Key NS. Inhibitors in congenital coagulation disorders. Br J Haematol 2004;127(4):379-91.
[4] Gren D. Factor VIII inhibitors: a 50-year perspective, Haemophilia 2011; 1–8.
[5] Green D, Lechner K. A survey of 215 nonhemophilic patients with inhibitors to factor VIII. Thromb Haemost 1981; 45: 200–3.
[6] Collins PW, Hirsch S, Baglin TP et al. Acquired hemophilia A in the United Kingdom: a 2-year national surveillance study by the United Kingdom Haemophilia Centre Doctors Organisation. Blood 2007; 109: 1870–7.
[7] Kim MS, Kilgore PE, Kang JS, Kim SY, Lee DY, Kim JS, Hwang PH.Transient acquired hemophilia associated with Mycoplasmapneumoniae pneumonia. J Korean Med Sci 2008 ; 23(1):138-41.
[8] Green D, Rademaker AW, Briet E. A prospective, randomized trial of prednisone and cyclophosphamide in the treatment of patients with factor VIII autoantibodies. Thromb Haemost 1993; 70: 753–7.
[9] Franchini M, Mannucci PM. Inhibitors of propagation of coagulation (factors VIII, IX and XI): a review of current therapeutic practice. Br J Clin Pharmacol 2011;72(4):553-62.
[10] Acharya SS, Coughlin A, Dimichele DM, North American Rare Bleeding Disorder Study Group. Rare Bleeding Disorder Registry: deficiencies of factors II, V, VII, X, XIII, fibrinogen and dysfibrinogenemias. J Thromb Haemost 2004;2(2):248-56.
[11] Wight J and Paisley S. The epidemiology of inhibitors in haemophilia A: a systematic review. Haemophilia 2003; 9, 418–435.

[12] Kempton CL, Soucie JM, Abshire TC. Incidence of inhibitors in a cohort of 838 males with hemophilia A previously treated with factor VIII concentrates. J ThrombHaemost. 2006;4 (12):2576-81.

[13] Lorenzo JI, López A, Altisent C, Aznar JA. Incidence of factor VIII inhibitors in severe haemophilia: the importance of patient age. Br J Haematol 2001;113(3):600-3.

[14] Chambost H. Assessing risk factors: prevention of inhibitors in haemophilia. Haemophilia 2010; 16 (Suppl. 2), 10–15

[15] Oldenburg J, El-Maarri O, Schwaab R. Inhibitor development in correlation to factor VIII genotypes. Haemophilia 2002; 8 (Suppl 2): 23–9.

[16] Oldenburg J, Brackmann HH, Schwaab R. Risk factors for inhibitor development in hemophilia A. Haematologica 2000; 85, (Suppl10):7-13; discussion 13-4.

[17] Oldenburg J, Schröder J, Brackmann HH, Möler-Reible C, Schwaab R, Tuddenham E. Environmental and genetic factors influencing inhibitor development. Semin Hematol 2004; 1(Suppl 1): 82–8.

[18] Schwaab R, Brackmann HH, Meyer C, Seehafer J, Kirchgesser M, Haack A, Olek K, Tuddenham EG, Oldenburg J.Haemophilia A: mutation type determines risk of inhibitor formation. Thromb Haemost 1995;74(6):1402-6.

[19] Oldenburg J, Schröder J, Schmitt C, Brackmann HH, Schwaab R. Small deletion/ insertion mutations within poly-A-runs of the factor VIII gene mitigate the severe haemophilia A phenotype. Thromb Haemost 1998; 79: 452-3.

[20] Warrier I. Data presented at the meeting of the Factor VIII and Factor IX Scientific Subcommittee of the SSC of the ISTH. 49th Annual Scientific and Standardization Committee meeting, Birmingham, UK, 2003. Available at: http://www.med.unc.edu/isth/; accessed 22 September 2004.

[21] Astermark J, Berntorp E, White GC, Kroner BL; MIBS Study Group. The Malmö International Brother Study (MIBS): further support for genetic predisposition to inhibitor development in hemophilia patients. Haemophilia 2001; 7: 267–72.

[22] Hay CR, Ollier W, Pepper L, Cumming A, Keeney S, Goodeve AC, Colvin BT, Hill FG, Preston FE, Peake IR. HLA class II profile: a weak determinant of factor VIII inhibitor development in severe haemophilia A. UKHCDO Inhibitor Working Party. Thromb Haemost 1997; 77: 234–7.

[23] Astermark J, Oldenburg J, Pavlova A, Berntorp E, Lefvert AK. Polymorphisms in the IL10 but not in the IL1beta and IL4 genes are associated with inhibitor development in patients with hemophilia A. Blood 2006; 107: 3167–72.

[24] Astermark J,Oldenburg J,Carlson J,Pavlova A,Kavakli K,Berntorp E, Lefvert AK. Polymorphisms in the TNFA gene and the risk of inhibitor development in patients with hemophilia A. Blood 2006; 108: 3739–45.

[25] Astermark J, Wang X, Oldenburg J, Berntorp E, Lefvert AK. Polymorphisms in the CTLA-4 gene and inhibitor development in patients with severe hemophilia A. J Thromb Haemost 2007; 5: 263– 5.

[26] Wieland I, Wermes C, Eifrig B et al. Inhibitor-Immunology-Study. Different HLA-types seem to be involved in the inhibitor development in haemophilia A. Hamostaseologie 2008; 28 (Suppl 1): S26–8.

[27] Viel KR, Ameri A, Abshire TC, Iyer RV, Watts RG, Lutcher C, Channell C, Cole SA, Fernstrom KM, Nakaya S, Kasper CK, Thompson AR, Almasy L, Howard TE

Inhibitors of factor VIII in black patients with hemophilia. N Engl J Med 2009;16;3 60(16):1618-27. Erratum in: N Engl J Med. 2009 Jul 30;361(5):544.
[28] Goudemand J, Rothschild C, Demiguel V et al. Influenceof the type of factor VIII concentrate on theincidence of factor VIII inhibitors in previously untreatedpatients with severe hemophilia A. Blood 2006;107: 46–51.
[29] Rasi V, Ikkala E. Haemophiliacs with factor VIII inhibitors in Finland: prevalence, incidence and outcome. Br J Haematol 1990;76(3):369-71.
[30] Shirahata A, Fukutake K, Higasa S, Mimaya J, Oka T, Shima M, Takamatsu J, Taki M, Taneichi M, Yoshioka A; STUDY GROUP ON FACTORS INVOLVED IN FORMATION OF INHIBITORS TO FACTOR VIII AND IX PREPARATIONS An analysis of factors affecting the incidence of inhibitor formation in patients with congenital haemophilia in Japan. Haemophilia 2011; 17(5): 771-6.
[31] Wang XF, Zhao YQ, Yang RC, et al. The prevalence of factorVIII inhibitors and genetic aspects of inhibitor developmentin Chinese patients with haemophilia A. Haemophilia 2010;16:632-9.
[32] Owaidah T and Al Momeen A. The first report of the Saudi national screening program for factor VIII and IX hemophila inhibitors. J Thromb Haemost 2011; 9, Suppl 2, 1-970. P-WE-132
[33] Gouw SC, van der Bom JG, AuerswaldG, et al. Recombinant versus plasma-derived factor VIII products and the development of inhibitors in previously untreated patients with severe hemophilia A: the CANAL cohort study. Blood 2007; 109: 4693–7.
[34] Lorenzo JI, Lopez A, Altisent C, Aznar JA. Incidence offactor VIII inhibitors in severe haemophilia: theimportance of patient age. Br J Haematol 2001; 113:600–3.
[35] Van der Bom JG, Mauser-Bunschoten EP, Fischer K,van den Berg HM. Age at first treatment and immunetolerance to factor VIII in severe hemophilia. ThrombHaemost 2003; 89: 475–9.
[36] Santagostino E, Mancuso ME, Rocino A et al. Environmentalrisk factors for inhibitor development inchildren with haemophilia A: a case-control study. Br J Haematol 2005; 130: 422–7.
[37] Gouw SC, van der Bom JG, Marijke van den Berg H.Treatment-related risk factors of inhibitor development in previously untreated patients with hemophilia A: the CANAL cohort study. Blood 2007; 109: 4648–54.
[38] Chalmers EA, Brown SA, Keeling D et al. Early factorVIII exposure and subsequent inhibitor development in children with severe haemophilia A. Haemophilia 2007; 13: 149–55.
[39] Gouw SC, van derBom JG, Marijke van den Berg H.Treatment-related risk factors of inhibitor development in previously untreated patients with hemophilia A: the CANAL cohort study. Blood 2007;109(11):4648-54.
[40] Gouw SC, van den Berg HM, le Cessie S, van der Bom JG. Treatment characteristics and the risk of inhibitordevelopment: a multicenter cohort study among previouslyuntreated patients with severe hemophilia A. J Thromb Haemost 2007; 5: 1383–90.
[41] Sharathkumar A, Lillicrap D, Blanchette VS et al.Intensive exposure to factor VIII is a risk factor forinhibitor development in mild hemophilia A. J Thromb Haemost 2003; 1: 1228–36.

[42] Schwarzinger I, Pabinger I, Korninger C, Haschke F, Kundi M, Niessner H, Lechner K. Incidence of inhibitorsin patients with severe and moderate hemophiliaA treated with factor VIII concentrates. Am J Hematol 1987; 24: 241–5.

[43] Lorenzo JI, Garcia R, Molina R. Factor VIII and Factor IX inhibitors in haemophiliacs. Lancet 1992; 339: 1550–1.

[44] Addiego J, Kasper C, Abildgaard C et al. Frequency of inhibitor development in haemophiliacs treated with low-purity factor VIII. Lancet 1993; 342: 462–464

[45] Schimpf K, Schwarz P, Kunschak M. Zero incidence of inhibitors in previously untreated patients who received intermediate purity factor VIII concentrate or factor IX complex. Thromb Haemost 1995; 73: 553–555.

[46] Guerois C, Laurian Y, Rothschild C et al. Incidence of factor VIII inhibitor development in severe hemophilia A patients treated only with one brand of highly purified plasma-derived concentrate. Thromb Haemost 1995; 73: 215–218.

[47] Addiego JR, Gomperts E, Liu SL, et al. Treatment of hemophilia with a highly purified factor VIII concentrate prepared by immunoaffinity chromatography. Thromb Haemost 1992; 67:19-27.

[48] Hoyer LW. Hemophilia A.N Engl J Med. 1994; 330 (1):38-47.

[49] Yee TT, Williams MD, Hill FGH, Lee CA, Pasi KJ.Absence of inhibitors in previously untreated patients with severe haemophilia A after exposure to a single intermediate purity factor VIII product.Thromb Haemost. 1997;78:1027-29.

[50] Dmoszynska A, Kuliczkowski K, Hellmann A, Trelinski J, Kloczko J, Baglin T, Hay C, O'Shaughnessy D, Zawilska K, Makris M, Shaikh-Zaidi R, Gascoigne E, Dash C. Clinical assessment of Optivate®, a high-purity concentrate of factor VIII with von Willebrand factor, in the management of patients with haemophilia A. Haemophilia. 2011;17(3):456-62.

[51] Klukowska A, Komrska V, Jansen M, Laguna P. Low incidence of factor VIII inhibitors in previously untreated patients during prophylaxis, on-demand treatment and surgical procedures, with Octanate®: interim report from an ongoing prospective clinical study. Haemophilia 2011;17(3): 399-406.

[52] Franchini M, Lippi G. Von Willebrand factor-containing factor VIII concentrates and inhibitors in haemophilia A. A critical literature review. ThrombHaemost. 2010;104 (5):931-40.

[53] Lusher JM, Arkin S, Abildgaard CF, Schwartz RS. Recombinant factor VIII for the treatment of previously untreated patients with hemophilia A. Safety, efficacy, and development of inhibitors. Kogenate Previously Untreated Patient Study Group. N Engl J Med 1993; 328: 453–459.

[54] Rothschild C, Laurian Y, Satre EP et al. French previously untreated patients with severe hemophilia A after exposure to recombinant factor VIII: incidence of inhibitor and evaluation of immune tolerance. Thromb Haemost 1998; 80: 779–783.

[55] Courter SG, Bedrosian CL. Clinical evaluation of B-domain deleted recombinant factor VIII in previously untreated patients. Semin Hematol 2001; 38: 52–59.

[56] Kreuz W, Gill JC, Rothschild C et al. Full-length sucrose-formulated recombinant factor VIII for treatment of previously untreated or minimally treated young children with severe haemophilia A: results of an international clinical investigation. Thromb Haemost 2005; 93: 457–467.

[57] Iorio A, Halimeh S, Holzhauer S, et al. Rate of inhibitor development in previously untreated hemophilia A patients treated with plasma-derived or recombinant factor VIII concentrates: a systematic review. J Thromb Haemost 2010 ;8(6):1256-65.
[58] Franchini M, Tagliaferri A, Mengoli C, Cruciani M. Cumulative inhibitor incidence in previously untreated patients with severe hemophilia A treated with plasma-derived versus recombinant factor VIII concentrates: A critical systematic review. Crit Rev Oncol Hematol 2011; *Available online 31 January 2011*
[59] Poon MC, Lillicrap D, Hensman C, Card R, Scully MF.Recombinant factor IX recovery and inhibitor safety: a Canadian post-licensure surveillance study. Thromb Haemost 2002; 87(3):431-5.
[60] Mannucci PM, Gringeri A, Peyvandi F, Factor VIII products and inhibitor development: the SIPPET study (survey of inhibitors in plasma-product exposed toddlers). Haemophilia 2007;13 (Suppl 5) :65-8.
[61] Mannucci P, Gringeri A, Peyvandi F, Santagostino E. Factor VIII products and inhibitor development: the SIPPET study (survey of inhibitors in plasma-product exposed toddlers). Haemophilia 2009; 13: 65–8.
[62] Gouw SC, ter Avest PC, van Helden PM, Voorberg J, van den Berg HM. Discordant antibody response in monozygotic twins with severe haemophilia A caused by intensive treatment. Haemophilia 2009; 15: 712–7.
[63] Gouw SC, van den Berg HM, le Cessie S, van der Bom JG. Treatment characteristics and the risk of inhibitor development: a multicenter cohort study among previously untreated patients with severe hemophilia A. J Thromb Haemost 2007; 5: 1383–90.
[64] Kempton CL.Inhibitors in previously treated patients: a review of the literature. Haemophilia 2010;16 (102):61-5.
[65] White GC, DiMichele D, Mertens K et al. Utilization of previously treated patients (PTPs), noninfected patients (NIPs), and previously untreated patients (PUPs) in the evaluation of new factor VIII and factor IX concentrates. Recommendation of the Scientific Subcommittee on Factor VIII and Factor IX of the Scientific and Standardization Committee of the International Society on Thrombosis and Haemostasis. Thromb Haemost 1999; 81: 462.
[66] Giles AR, Rivard GE, Teitel J, Walker I. Surveillance for factor VIII inhibitor development in the Canadian Hemophilia A population following the widespread introduction of recombinant factor VIII replacement therapy. Transfus Sci 1998; 19: 139–48.
[67] Peerlinck K, Arnout J, Di Giambattista M et al. Factor VIII inhibitors in previously treated haemophilia A patients with adouble virus-inactivated plasma derived factor VIII concentrate. Thromb Haemost 1997; 77: 80–6.
[68] Peerlinck K, Arnout J, Gilles JG, Saint-Remy JM, Vermylen J. A higher than expected incidence of factor VIII inhibitors in multitransfusedhaemophilia A patients treated with an intermediate purity pasteurized factor VIII concentrate. Thromb Haemost 1993; 69: 115–18.
[69] Rosendaal FR, Nieuwenhuis HK, van den Berg HM et al. A sudden increase in factor VIII inhibitor development in multitransfused hemophilia A patients in the Netherlands. Dutch Hemophilia Study Group. Blood 1993; 81: 2180–6.
[70] Giles AR, Rivard GE, Teitel J, Walker I. Surveillance for factorVIII inhibitor development in the Canadian Hemophilia A populationfollowing the widespread

introduction of recombinantfactor VIII replacement therapy. Transfus Sci 1998; 19: 139–48.

[71] Rubinger M, Lillicrap D, Rivard GE et al. A prospective surveillance study of factor VIII inhibitor development in the Canadian haemophiliaA population following the switch to a recombinantfactor VIII product formulated with sucrose. Haemophilia 2008;14: 281–6.

[72] Vidovic N, Musso R, Klamroth R, Enriquez MM, Achilles K Postmarketing surveillance study of KOGENATE Bayer with Bio-Set in patients with haemophilia A: evaluation of patients' satisfaction after switch to the new reconstitution system. Haemophilia 2010 16(1):66-71. Biggs R, Bidwell E. A method for the studyof antihaemophilic globulin inhibitors withreference to six cases. Br J Haematol 1959;5: 379–95.

[73] Kasper CK, Aledort LM, Counts RB et al. A more uniform measurement of factor VIII inhibitors. Thrombdiath Haemorrh 1975;34: 869–72

[74] Verbruggen B, Novakova I, Wessels H,Boezeman J, van den Berg M, Mauser-Bunshoten E. The Nijmegen modification of the Bethesda assay for factor VIII:C inhibitors: improved specificity and reliability. Thromb Haemost 1995; 73: 247–51.

[75] Giles AR, Verbruggen B, Rivard GE, Teitel J, Walker. A detailed comparison of the performance of the standard versus the Nijmegen modification of the Bethesda assay in detecting factor VIII:C inhibitors in the haemophilia A population of Canada. Association of Hemophilia Centre Directors of Canada. Factor VIII/IX Subcommittee of Scientific and Standardization Committee of International Society on Thrombosis and Haemostasis. Thromb Haemost 1998;79(4):872-5.

[76] Verbruggen B, Giles A, Samis J, Verbeek K, Mensink E, Nováková I. The type of factor VIII deficient plasma used influences the performance of the Nijmegen modification of the Bethesda assay for factor VIII inhibitors. Thromb Haemost. 2001; 86(6):1435-9.

[77] Sahud MA, Pratt KP, Zhukov O, Qu K, Thompson AR. ELISA system for detection of immune responses to FVIII: a study of 246 samples and correlation with the Bethesda assay. Haemophilia 2007;13(3):317-22.

[78] Owaidah T, Nasr R and Al Moomn A. Comparison between ELISA based test for detection of factor VIII antibodies screen and standard Bethesda. J Thromb Haemost 2011; 9, Suppl 2: 1-970 P-WE-212.

[79] Zakarija A, Harris S, Rademaker AW, Brewer J, Krudysz-Amblo J, Butenas S, Mann KG, Green D. Alloantibodies to factor VIII in haemophilia. Haemophilia 2011;17(4):636-40.

6

Prospective Efficacy and Safety of a Novel Bypassing Agent, FVIIa/FX Mixture (MC710) for Hemophilia Patients with Inhibitors

Kazuhiko Tomokiyo, Yasushi Nakatomi,
Takayoshi Hamamoto and Tomohiro Nakagaki
Therapeutic Protein Product Research Department
The Chemo-Sero-Therapeutic Research Institute, Kaketsuken
Japan

1. Introduction

Hemophilia A and B are hereditary bleeding disorders caused by a deficiency of coagulation factors VIII (FVIII) and IX (FIX), respectively. In substitution therapies using FVIII and FIX concentrates for the management of bleeding, the development of inhibitory antibodies is a serious complication in ~28% and ~7% of hemophilia A and B patients, respectively **[1, 2]**.
Currently, two bypassing agents, plasma-derived activated prothrombin complex concentrates (APCC, FEIBA®) and recombinant activated factor VII (rFVIIa, NovoSeven®), are available for the management of bleeding in hemophilia patients with inhibitors including acquired hemophilia patients. Retrospective studies showed the efficacy of rFVIIa and APCC in 12~36 h in a standard administration regime is assessed to be 66~95% and 39~76%, respectively **[3]**. A recent comparative study seemed to indicate equivalence between rFVIIa and APCC **[4]**; however, a considerable number of patients experience treatment failure or insufficient efficacy.
In 2002, an anecdotal report suggested that the sequential administration of rFVIIa and prothrombin complex concentrate (PCC) to hemophilia patients with inhibitors in order to obtain a stronger hemostatic effect than with rFVIIa alone **[5]**. Further, it has been reported that the combination of rFVIIa and APCC appeared to confer beneficial hemostatic synergy in patients refractory to each individual therapy **[6-8]**. However, repeated infusion of APCC may cause an accumulation of prothrombin and factor X (FX), thereby increasing the risk of thrombosis. Moreover, a lack of suitable laboratory tests for monitoring hemostatic effects is a major concern with current bypassing therapies. As a consequence and in appreciation of the incomplete efficacy and safety of currently available bypassing agents, new drugs are in development, such as rFVIIa analogues featuring higher hemostatic potential **[9]**, glycoPEGylated rFVIIa with a longer half-life than rFVIIa **[10]**, and non-anticoagulant sulphated polysaccharides (AV513) **[11]**.
In order to solve these problems, we searched for alternative factors for enhancing and promoting FVIIa's hemostatic activity, and found that a combination of plasma-derived FVIIa and FX (FVIIa/FX) may overcome the disadvantages of rFVIIa therapy for hemophilia patients with inhibitors. That combination allows improving APTT remarkably in the

patient plasma which is useful laboratory test for monitoring the hemostatic effect of hemophilia patients. An FVIIa/FX mixture, MC710, was designed as a dry-heated product prepared by mixing plasma-derived FVIIa and FX at a weight ratio of 1:10 under acidic conditions to suppress the generation of FXa.

A Phase I clinical study encompassing pharmacokinetics (PK), pharmacodynamics (PD), and safety has been completed. In this article, we outline the rationale for the combined use of FVIIa and FX, the manufacturing method of MC710, the treatment's prospective efficacy and safety, and in the final section, the results of Phase I clinical study in non-bleeding hemophilia patients with inhibitors.

2. Rationale for the combination of FVIIa and FX

2.1 Background

The blood coagulation system involves a so-called "cascade reaction" of enzymes and substrates which finally achieves the formation of a fibrin clot. In this reaction, Ca^{2+} and phosolipids (PL) assume the role of cofactors which remarkably enhance the affinity between enzymes and substrates, resulting in the promotion of a coagulation reaction at the site of injury.

FVIIa circulates in blood at a concentration of around 0.1 nM (3~5 ng mL^{-1}) in plasma **[12, 13]** with a much longer half life, 2~3 h, than other activated coagulation factors because of its zymogen-like conformation **[14]**. Tissue factor (TF) is a membrane glycoprotein expressed in various tissues and plays the role of a cofactor of FVIIa. Vascular TF is present in the adventitia, hidden from the circulating blood. When a vessel is injured, TF is exposed at the site. FVIIa binds to TF forming a stoichiometric complex (the initiator of the extrinsic pathway) and remarkably enhances catalytic activity to activate FIX and FX. FIXa forms a FIXa/FVIIIa/PL complex (FXase) and converts FX to FXa. Also, FXa forms a FXa/FVa/PL complex (prothrombinase) and converts prothrombin to thrombin. Thrombin activates FXI to form FXIa and promotes the activation of FIX (feedback activation of the intrinsic pathway), and converts the fibrinogen to a fibrin clot via limited proteolysis **[15]**. Platelets are essential for hemostasis. In the artery, circulating platelets in blood attach and adhere to the extracellular matrix (collagen) under the layer of endothelial cells at the site of damage using GPVI and integrin $\alpha_2\beta_1$ (GPIa/IIa), and adhere to the collagen via the interaction of VWF (von Willebrand factor) and GPIbIX, and finally aggregate through the interaction of $\alpha_{IIb}\beta_3$ (GPIIb/IIIa) and VWF/fibrinogen **[16-19]**. Through these processes, localized platelets are activated by thrombin or chemical mediators (ADP, *et al*) released from activated platelet granules. The PL membrane essential for thrombin generation is mainly supplied by the activated platelets.

In the hemostasis of hemophilia patients with inhibitors against FIX or FVIII, the intrinsic pathway is completely blocked. Therefore, it is necessary to enhance the potential for coagulation based on the extrinsic pathway, the activation of FX by FVIIa, followed by the activation of prothrombin to form thrombin.

In 1996, rFVIIa therapy was launched to give a super-physiological concentration to the patient plasma to enhance the extrinsic pathway of hemophilia patients with inhibitors. However, the mechanism of the bypassing activity of rFVIIa is controversial due to the requirement for a high dose (60~120 μg kg^{-1}), which gives a high FVIIa concentration in plasma (0.5~1.0 μg mL^{-1}) **[20]**.

There are two hypotheses to elucidate the requirement for the high dose **(Fig. 1-A)**. The first is "TF-dependent FX activation". It was reported that rFVIIa-induced thrombin generation in the presence of a low concentration of TF and in the absence of FVIII is inhibited by physiological concentrations of FVII, and at least 10 nM (0.5 μg mL^{-1}) of rFVIIa is required to overcome the inhibition by FVII in order to induce the bypassing activity **[21, 22].** The second is "TF-independent FX activation". It was reported that 5 nM (0.25 μg mL^{-1}) of rFVIIa could convert FX to FXa on the surface of activated platelets, leading to thrombin generation independent of TF **[23]**. Clinical experience has suggested that the dose or blood level of rFVIIa required for hemostasis in any given hemophilia patient with inhibitors is not always predictable. Differences in platelet procoagulant properties could influence the response to a high-dose of rFVIIa **[24, 25]**. Also, it has been reported that rFVIIa binds to GPIbIX on activated platelets and localizes at the site of injury **[26]**. Recently, mega-dose therapy with an injection of rFVIIa (270 μg kg^{-1}) has been applied to the control of bleeding to diminish repeated administrations in 2~3 h and raise the hemostatic potential of rFVIIa by increasing the C_{max} in plasma above the standard dose **[27, 28]**.
The exact mechanism of rFVIIa is not clear at present, but its potential for FXa and thrombin generation and subsequent fibrin clot formation will be essential to obtain a hemostatic effect with rFVIIa, in either a TF-dependent or TF-independent manner.

2.2 Rationale for the combined use of FVIIa and FX

It was reported that TF binds to FX or FIX as well as to FVIIa and this ternary complex of enzyme/cofactor/substrate (FVIIa/TF/ FIX or FX) is the real trigger of the extrinsic pathway to generating FIXa or FXa and the subsequent generation of thrombin **[29-31]**. However, it was demonstrated that FIX is a much better substrate for FVIIa-TF than FX **[32]**. We investigated the kinetic parameters of FVIIa-mediated FX activation under several conditions. The results of the kinetic analysis are shown in **Table 1.** K_m values in the presence of PL and relipidated TF were 180 ± 70 nM and 160 ± 60 nM, while k_{cat} values were 0.38 ± 0.09 s^{-1} and 11.5 ± 4.7 s^{-1}, respectively, similar to values published previously **[32]**. The FX level in normal plasma is 8~12 μg mL^{-1} (140~210 nM) **[34],** and the K_m values were within this range; therefore, it was suggested that the FX concentration in plasma might not be sufficient to achieve the generation of FXa by FVIIa required for hemostasis **(Fig. 1-B)**. These results indicate that a higher concentration of FX is required to enhance the catalytic efficacy of FVIIa and to complete coagulation in the plasma of hemophilia patients.

Assay conditions	Concentration	K_m μM	k_{cat} s^{-1}	k_{cat}/K_m s^{-1} μM^{-1}
Ca^{2+}	5 mM	72.4	0.000135	0.00000187
Ca^{2+}/PCPS[a)]	5 mM/10 μM	0.18±0.07	0.38±0.09	2.20±0.34
Ca^{2+}/PCPS/TF	5 mM/10 μM/100 pM	0.16±0.06	11.5±4.7	73.1±14.3
Ca^{2+}/activated platelets[b)]	5 mM/1.5×10^5 cells μL^{-1}	1.72±0.4	0.77±0.21	0.48±0.19

The activation of FX was carried out in the presence or absence of PL (10 μM) and relipidated TF (100 pM TF/10 μM PL) in a solution containing 5 mM $CaCl_2$ **[33]**.
a) Reconstituted phosphatidylcholine and phosphatidylserine vesicles (PCPS; weight ratio 7:3) were used as phospholipids.
b) Platelets were activated by the thrombin receptor activation peptide (TRAP).

Table 1. Steady-state kinetics of FX's activation by FVIIa

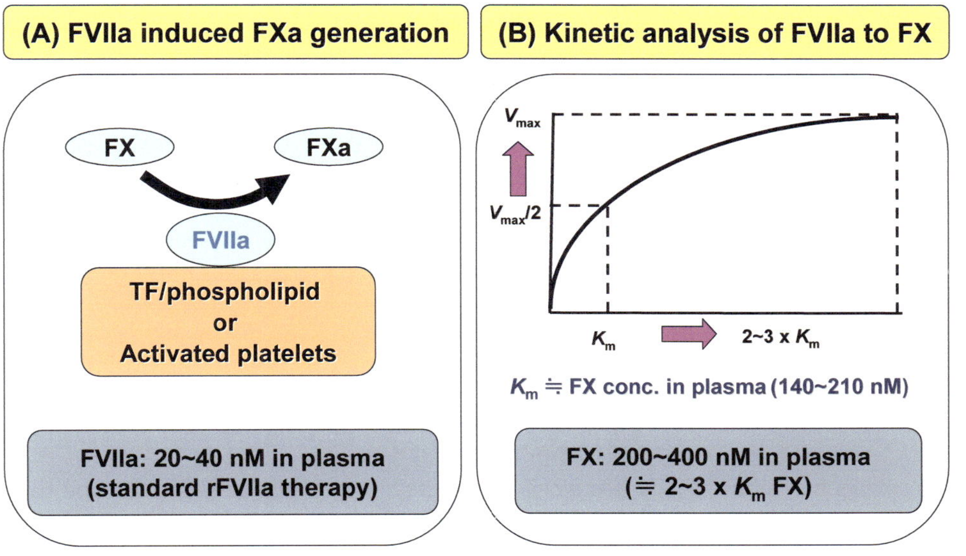

(A) FVIIa induced FXa generation. The activation of FX is essential for FVIIa to generate bypassing activity. For the elucidation of the requirement for high rFVIIa concentrations (>1 µg mL^{-1} in plasma) in rFVIIa therapy, there are two hypotheisies: "TF-dependent FX activation" **[21, 22]** and "TF-independent FX activation" **[23-26] (refer to the text for details).** (B) Kinetic analysis of FVIIa to FX. In the activation of FX by FVIIa, the activation rate (y-axis) increases depending on the substrate (FX) concentration (x-axis). As shown in **Table 1,** K_m values in the presence of PL and relipidated TF were in the range of FX levels in normal plasma (140~210 nM), and the K_m value in activated platelets is far above that range. In the extrinsic pathway, the increase of FX concentration in plasma two or three times (2~3 x K_m) might facilitate the increase of the FX actvation rate, and promote the formation of FVIIa/TF/FX complex.

Fig. 1. Advantage of co-administration of FVIIa and FX

The results of the kinetic analysis were consistent with those of the thrombin generation (TG) assay **(Fig. 2)**. TG assay using a fluorosubstrate (Z-G-G-R-MCA) specific for thrombin was developed by Hemker et al **[35]**. In this assay system, thrombin generation is analyzed in the following three steps **[36, 37]**:

1. Initiation: initiation of the cascade reaction to start thrombin generation.
2. Propagation: explosive thrombin production.
3. Termination: attenuation of thrombin generation.

The TG assay is used to analyze the clinical efficacy of rFVIIa and APCC **[38].** The TG parameters are lag time (time to initial thrombin formation (min)), peak thrombin level (nM), time to peak (ttPeak) (min), and endogenous thrombin potential (ETP) (nM min) **[39]**. We used this assay to examine the hemostatic potential of the combination of FVIIa and FX. The thrombin-generating potential of hemophilic plasma was raised by increasing the concentration of FX added to the plasma in the range of 2.5~20 µg mL^{-1} without the addition of FVIIa **(Figs. 2A-a and 2B-a)**. Further, the combination of FVIIa (0.25 and 1.0 µg mL^{-1}) and FX (2.5~20 µg mL^{-1}) gave more thrombin-generating potential to the plasma than did FVIIa alone, resulting in a shortening of the ttPeak and an increase in the peak thrombin level **(Figs. 2A-b and -c, and 2B-b and -c) [40]**.
It has been estimated that the half-life of FVIIa is around 3 h and that of FX is 24~56 h **[41-43]**. Following the simultaneous administration of FVIIa and FX, the amount of FVIIa should

decrease faster than that of FX, but a high FX level might help to generate bypassing activity which results in longer-lasting hemostatic potential than FVIIa alone. This idea was proven in our previous experiment using a monkey acquired hemophilia B model in which the hemostatic efficacy of FVIIa/FX (co-administration of FVIIa (80 μg kg^{-1}) and FX (800 μg kg^{-1})) and FVIIa alone (80 μg kg^{-1}) was compared by measuring thromboelastography (TEG). As shown in **Fig. 3**, administration of FVIIa/FX remarkably normalized TEG parameters. Even 6 h after its administration, FVIIa/FX had hemostatic potential above that immediately after the administration of FVIIa alone **[44]**.

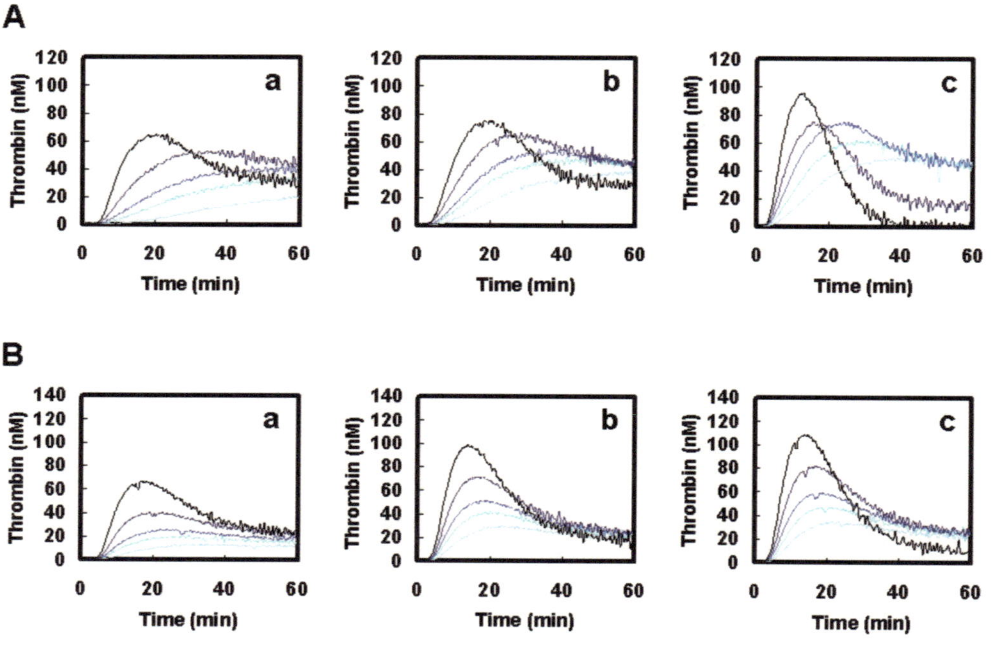

TG in plasma of a hemophilia A patient with inhibitors (FVIII INP; 101 BU mL^{-1}) or FIX-depleted plasma (FIX-DP) at various concentrations of FVIIa and FX with relipidated TF. Panels a~c of A (FVIII INP) and B (FIX-DP): FVIIa 0, 0.25, and 1.0 μg mL^{-1}. Added FX concentration in the plasma from top to bottom in each panel: 0 μg mL^{-1}, – ; 2.5 μg mL^{-1}, – ; 5.0 μg mL^{-1}, – ;10 μg mL^{-1}, – ;20 μg mL^{-1}, – . 16.7 pM TF and 0.83 μM PL were used for the assay.

Fig. 2. Changes in TG profiles induced by FX on FVIIa in hemophilic plasma(40)

APTT is used for monitoring the management of bleeding or determining the supplemental level of FVIII or FIX concentrate in hemophilia patients, but not in therapy using bypassing agents because of the poor improvement. We reported that more than 5 μg mL^{-1} of FVIIa alone is required to reduce APTT in hemophilic plasma to levels equivalent to those after replacement-therapy (10 % of FVIII or FIX activity in hemophilic plasma); on the other hand, the mixture of FX and FVIIa caused a significant improvement of APTT in a concentration-dependent manner. In plasma containing 0.5~1.5 μg mL^{-1} of FVIIa (obtained after intravenous rFVIIa administration at standard doses) when FX is added at 5~15 μg mL^{-1}, the poor coagulant activity in hemophilic plasma is remarkably improved to levels achieved

with replacement therapy **[44]**. Therefore, a mixture ratio 1: 10 of FVIIa to FX in MC710 was designed to optimize the bypassing effect of FVIIa (0.5~1.5 μg mL^{-1}) in plasma.

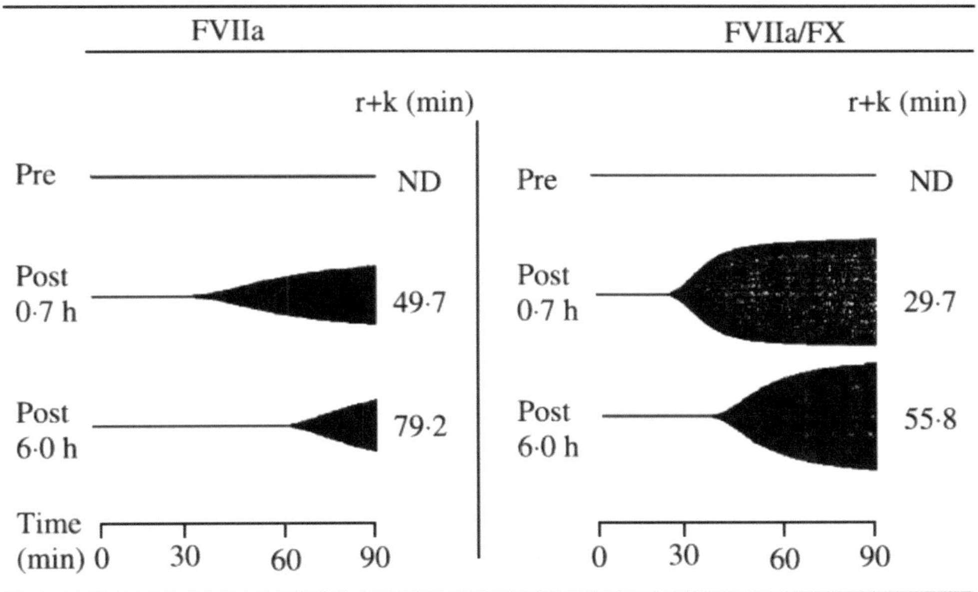

A hemophilia B model using a cynomolgus monkey was produced by the administration of goat anti-FIX antibodies to be in < 5% of FIX activity. FVIIa (80 μg/kg) was administered to the monkey and Thromboelastography (TEG) was measured pre-administration, and 6 h and 12 h post-administration. Also, FVIIa (80 μg/kg) and FX (800 μg/kg) were continuously injected into the monkey. The TEG patterns are shown in the figure and r + k values are described on the right side of each pattern. ND means "not detected".

Fig. 3. Changes in TEG patterns in the monkey acquired hemophilia B model pre/post injection of FVIIa or FVIIa/FX(44)

3. Outline of the manufacture of the FVIIa/FX mixture (MC710)

MC710 is a lyophilized mixture of FVIIa and FX prepared from pooled human plasma. FVII and FX are vitamin K-dependent proteins containing a strongly negatively charged amino acid, γ-carboxy-glutamic acid. The purification of those proteins takes into account specific properties such as high acidity and Ca^{2+}-dependent conformational change. The conversion of FVII to FVIIa is a key process in the production of the FVIIa preparation. In 1986, Bjoern *et al.* reported that rFVII is autocatalytically activated to rFVIIa on an anion exchange column **[45]**. On an industrial scale, the activation of FVII on an anion exchange resin is very useful because it does not require any other proteases to activate FVII such as FXa, FIXa, and FXIIa. In the production of plasma-derived FVIIa, FVII is converted to FVIIa with the following two steps to achieve high recovery and quality: (1) partial activation on anion exchange resin and, (2) further activation in the solution after eluting from the resin **[46]**. A flow diagram of the preparation of MC710 is shown in **Fig. 4**. In the first purification step, a crude

vitamin K-dependent protein fraction is extracted from cryoprecipitate-poor plasma using anion exchange chromatography. Next, this fraction is applied to an immunoaffinity chromatography column containing gels bound with Ca^{2+}-dependent anti-FVII or anti-FX monoclonal antibody as a ligand. The FVII or FX fraction eluted with a buffer containing EDTA is treated in solvent and detergent (0.3% TNBP and 1% polysorbate 80) for virus inactivation. After the treatment, the FVII fraction is applied to DEAE Sepharose-FF to obtain partially activated FVIIa and the eluted FVII/FVIIa mixture is completely converted to FVIIa in the solution. The FX fraction eluted from the immunoaffinity chromatography

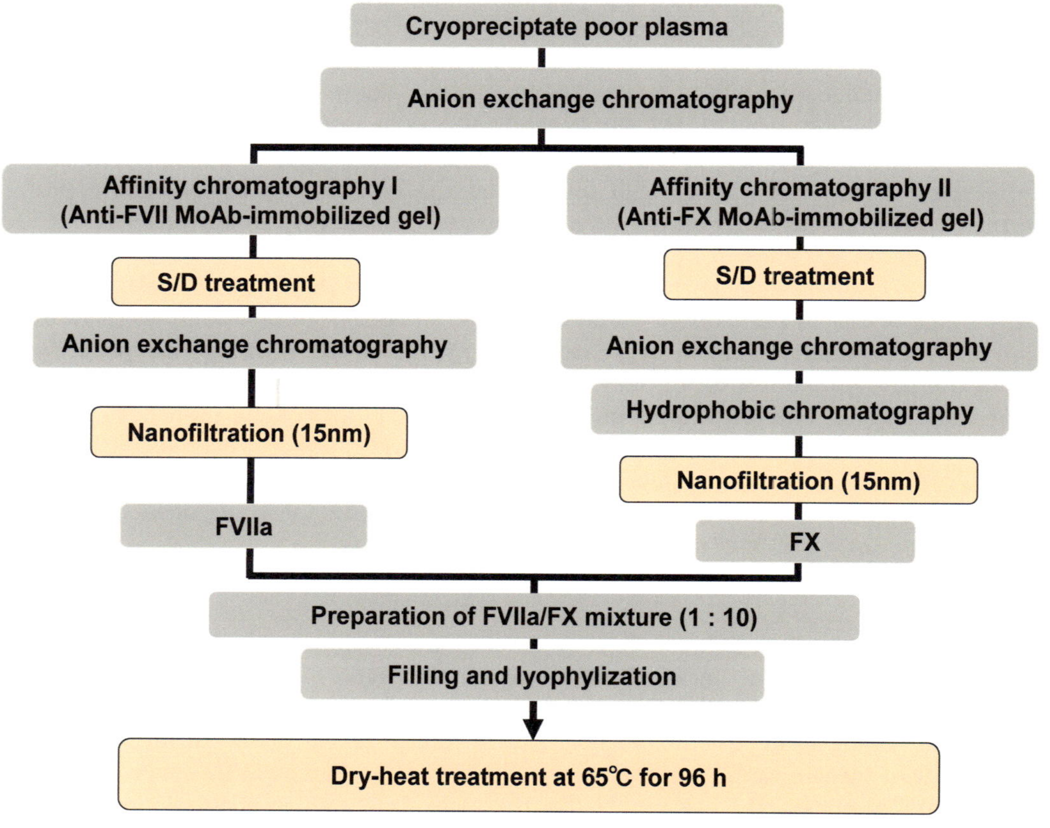

FVII and FX are purified using immunoaffinity gel coupled with anti- FVII and -FX antibodies, respectively. Purified fractions are treated with solvent and detergent (0.3% TNBP and 1% polysorbate 80) for inactivation of the enveloped virus, and purified samples are filtered with a nano-filter of 15-nm pore size (Planova® 15N) for virus elimination. The specific activity of the prepared FVIIa and FX was 48.1 ± 0.5 IU/µg (n=5) and 159.1 ± 4.4 IU/mg (n=6), respectively. After mixing FVIIa and FX with the stabilizers, the solution is dispensed to the vials and lyophilized, then heated at 65°C for 96 h.

Fig. 4. Outline of manufacturing methods of MC710

column is further purified using anion exchange and hydrophobic interaction chromatographies. These purified samples are filtered with a nano-filter (Planova® 15N) of 15-nm pore size for virus elimination. The concentrated FVIIa and FX are mixed at a weight ratio of 1:10 under acidic conditions of pH5.5~5.9 for suppression of FXa generation, and then lyophilized. Finally, the lyophilized FVIIa and FX mixture is dry-heated at 65°C for 96 h for virus elimination. MC710 is formulated with FVIIa (0.6 mg mL^{-1}), FX (6 mg mL^{-1}), antithrombin (1.0 U mL^{-1}), and human serum albumin (2.0%) after reconstitution **[40]**.

4. Prospective efficacy and safety of MC710

4.1 APTT and PT waveform analysis

APTT waveforms are used to analyze the overall process of fibrin clotting by measuring the turbidity and calculating the coagulation rate (dT/dt) and coagulation acceleration (second derivative of transmittance and time; d^2T/dt^2). It was reported that these parameters are useful for the diagnosis of DIC **[47, 48]**. Recently, Shima reported that APTT waveforms are applicable to the quantification of low levels of FVIII (<1 U dL^{-1}) on the basis of the correlation of the FVIII activity with coagulation acceleration, and the waveform profile formed by rFVIIa was different from that for normal plasma **[49]**. In our analysis, MC710 with a FVIIa concentration of 1 μg mL^{-1} (the dose and concentration in plasma of MC710 are expressed as FVIIa amounts) exhibited greater clotting ability than 1 μg mL^{-1} FVIIa alone in hemophilia A patient plasma with inhibitors and FIX-deficient plasma samples **(Figs. 5A-a and 5B-a).** Coagulation acceleration showed that MC710 at above 1-2 μg mL^{-1} possessed a greater ability to shorten APTT and to induce accelerated clotting than did the same concentration of rFVIIa **(Figs. 5A-b and 5B-b)**. Parameters for plasma from hemophilia A patients with inhibitors in the presence of 1 U mL^{-1} APCC were similar to those in the presence of 1 μg mL^{-1} MC710 **(Figs. 5A-a and 5A-b).** On the other hand, PT and its clot formation acceleration did not show any difference among the three agents **(data not shown)**.

4.2 TG assay

The thrombin generation of hemophilia A patient plasma with inhibitors and FIX-depleted plasma was measured at various concentrations of rFVIIa, MC710, and APCC. MC710 (0.1~8.0 μg mL^{-1}) and APCC (0.25~2.0 U mL^{-1}) exhibited conspicuous concentration-dependent changes in thrombin generation profiles **(Figs. 6A-b, 6B-b, and 7B-a)**. Reportedly, a mega-dose (270 μg kg^{-1} b.w.) of rFVIIa can achieve rFVIIa concentrations of 3~5 μg mL^{-1} in hemophilic plasma **[27, 28]**; however, the thrombin-generating potential of rFVIIa in plasma did not change at over 1 μg mL^{-1} of rFVIIa **(Figs. 6A-a and 6B-a)**.

To evaluate the TF-specificity of the agents, thrombin generation in plasma of a hemophilia patient with inhibitors was measured in the presence or absence of relipidated TF or PL at various concentrations of MC710 and APCC, and 1.0 μg mL^{-1} of rFVIIa **(Figs. 7A-a~c and 7Ba~c)**. The 0.1 μg mL^{-1} of MC710 and 0.25 U mL^{-1} of APCC showed a greater thrombin generation potential than 1.0 μg mL^{-1} of rFVIIa **(Figs. 7A-a and 7B-a).** MC710 showed lower thrombin-generating potential than did APCC in the absence of TF or PL **(Figs. 7A-b and -c, and 7B-b and -c)**. These results suggest that MC710 has a relatively high specificity for TF compared to APCC.

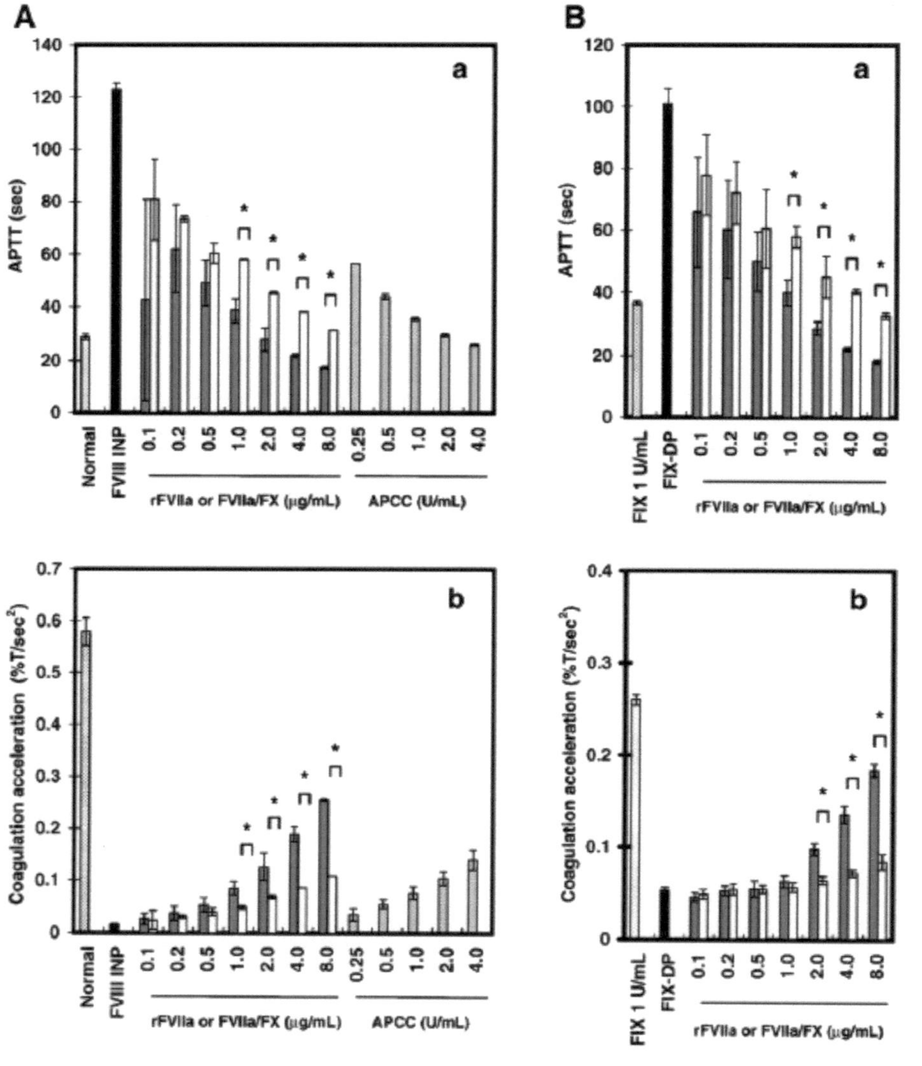

APTT waveforms of plasma from a hemophilia A patient with inhibitors (FVIII INP; 140 BU mL^{-1}) and FIX-depleted plasma (FIX-DP) at various concentrations of the bypassing agents. Panels A-a and A-b: APTT and coagulation acceleration of FVIII INP containing rFVIIa (NovoSeven®) (0.1~8.0 μg mL^{-1}, □), MC710 (0.1~8.0 μg mL^{-1}, ■), and APCC (FEIBA®) (0.25~4.0 U mL^{-1}). Panels B-a and B-b: APTT and coagulation acceleration of FIX-DP containing rFVIIa (0.1~8.0 μg mL^{-1}, □), MC710 (0.1~8.0 μg mL^{-1}, ■). Normal plasma ("Normal") or FIX-DP supplemented with FIX at 1 U mL^{-1} was used as a control. The MC710 concentration is denoted by the FVIIa concentration in each panel.

Fig. 5. Changes in APTT waveforms induced by rFVIIa, APCC, and MC710(40)

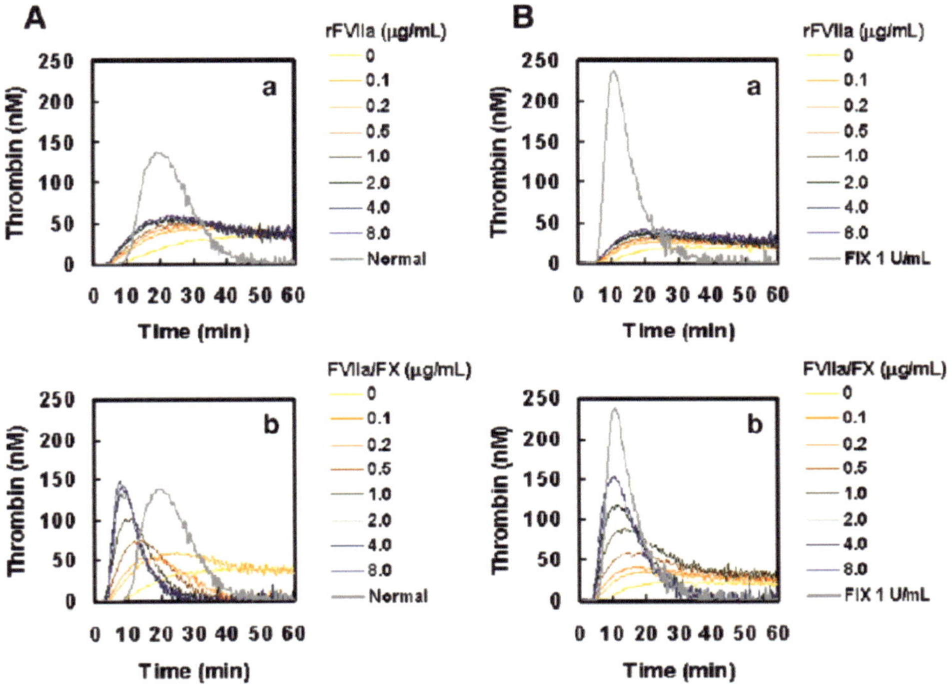

TG in plasma of a hemophilia A patient on inhibitors (FVIII INP; 70 BU mL^{-1}) and FIX-depleted plasma (FIX-DP) at various concentrations of the bypassing agents with relipidated TF. Panels A-a and -b: TG of FVIII INP; rFVIIa (NovoSeven®) (A-a, 0.1~8 µg mL^{-1}) and MC710 (A-b, 0.1~8.0 µg mL^{-1}). Panels B-a and -b: TG of FIX-DP, rFVIIa (B-a, 0.1~8.0 µg mL^{-1}), MC710 (B-b, 0.1~8.0 µg mL^{-1}). The gray lines signify the results in normal plasma ("Normal") for A-a and -b and FIX-DP supplemented with FIX 1.0 U mL^{-1} for B-a and B-b used as control plasma. The MC710 concentration is denoted by the FVIIa concentration in each panel. In the TG assay, 16.7 pM TF and 0.83 µM PL were used. Each TG profile represents the results of three experiments.

Fig. 6. Changes in TG profiles induced by rFVIIa and MC710(40)

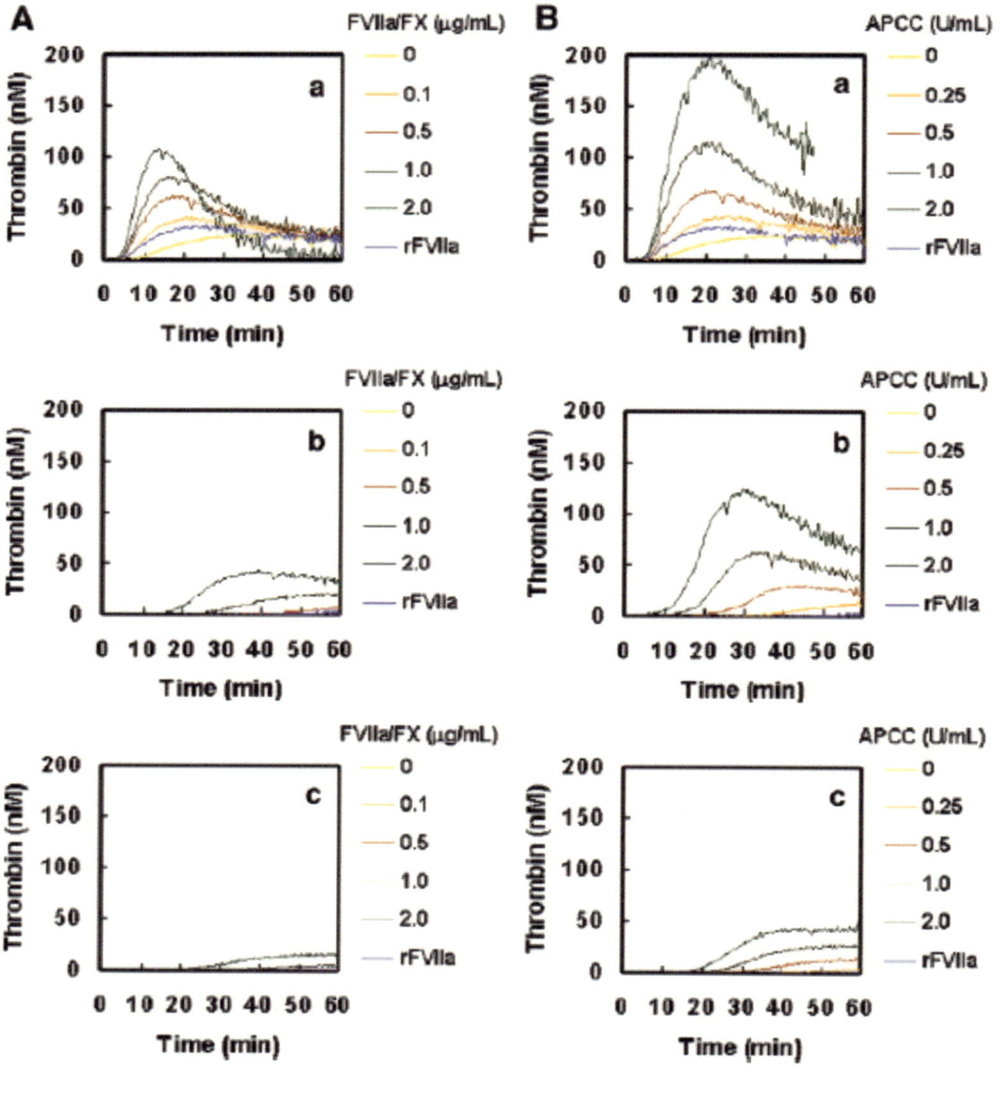

TG in plasma of a hemophilia A patient on inhibitors (38 BU mL^{-1}) with relipidated TF or phospholipids or without relipidated TF at various concentrations of the bypassing agents. Panels A- and B-a~c: a) addition of relipidated TF, b) addition of phospholipids, c) no addition of relipidated TF at the concentrations of MC710 (0.1~2.0 µg mL^{-1}; panels A a~c) and APCC (FEIBA®) (0.25-2.0 U mL^{-1}; panels B a~c). TG in the presence of rFVIIa (NovoSeven®) (1.0 µg mL^{-1}) is inserted in each panel. The MC710 concentration is denoted by the FVIIa concentration in each panel. Each TG profile represents the results of three experiments. In the TG assay, 16.7 pM TF and 0.83 µM PL were used.

Fig. 7. Changes in TG profiles induced by APCC and MC710 with or without TF(40)

4.3 Thrombogenic test using monkeys

It was reported that APCCs might induce thrombotic complications such as disseminated intravascular coagulation (DIC) and acute myocardial infarction **[50-52]**. As the clearance of FX is much slower than that of FVIIa, repeated administrations of MC710 might induce the accumulation of FX in the blood raising concerns over safety regarding DIC or other thrombotic events. Therefore, it is important to confirm the safety of repeated administrations of MC710 alone and in combination with other bypassing agents. We performed multiple injections of MC710 (4 injections of 120 μg kg^{-1} every 8 h (as FVIIa dose)), and rFVIIa (one injection of 90 μg kg^{-1} and 2 injections of 120 μg kg^{-1} every 2 h) or APCC (3 infusions of 100 U kg^{-1} every 12 h) at 8 h after the administration of MC710 (120 μg kg^{-1}) into the monkeys, and compared the DIC parameter changes with those of APCC (4 infusion of 100 U kg^{-1} every 12 h) **(Fig. 8)**. No serious or severe event was observed in any monkey or in any group, and the fibrinogen level and platelet counts did not change. However, the FDP (fibrinogen degraded products) level increased in all groups and the rate of increase was lower in the group repeatedly administered MC710 than that repeatedly administered APCC **(See the legend in Fig. 8).** These results suggest the thrombogenic risk from the repeated administration of MC710 is equal to or lower than that of repeated administration of APCC.

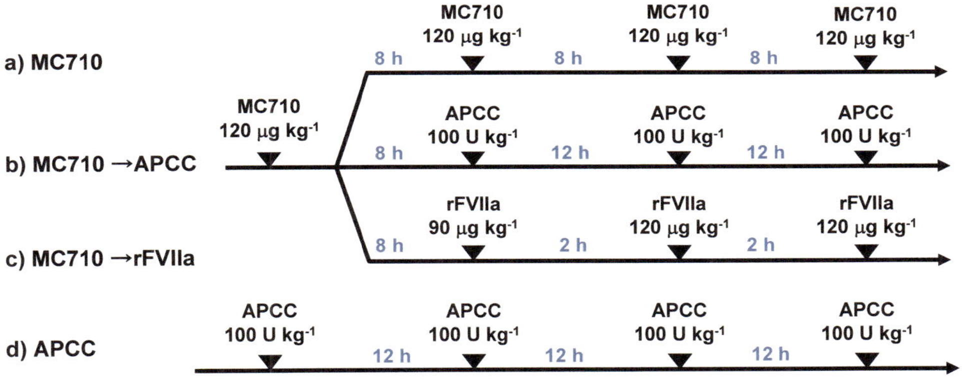

Thrombogenicity of MC710 was compared to APCC (FEIBA®) using cynomolgus monkeys. The experimental design is described in the figure. Schemes a)~c) show the time courses of injections or infusions of rFVIIa (NovoSeven®) and APCC after 120 μg $kg^{-1}$of MC710. MC710 dose is denoted as FVIa dose. Scheme d) shows the time course of repeated infusions of APCC. The experiment was performed using three monkeys in each group. At pre-administrations FDP level was 0.44 ± 0.24 ng mL^{-1} (n=12) and at 30 min after the final administration of the agents a), b), c), and d) were 3.37 ± 3.59, 5.87 ± 2.64, 2.93 ± 0.42, and 8.57 ± 2.17 ng mL^{-1} (n=3), respectively.

Fig. 8. Design for the thrombognenic test for MC710

5. Summary of phase I clinical study

5.1 Outline of the trial

Phase I clinical study of MC710 has been completed. In this study, PK and PD parameters and the safety of single doses of MC710 were investigated in 11 hemophilia patients with inhibitors in a non-bleeding state. A total of 25 administrations of MC710 were made to the subjects (7 hemophilia A patients with inhibitors and 4 hemophilia B patients with inhibitors) at 5 doses

of MC710 (20, 40, 80, 100 and 120 μg kg^{-1} (as FVIIa dose)) in addition to the administrations of rFVIIa 120 μg kg^{-1}, and APCC 50 U kg^{-1} or 75 U kg^{-1} as active controls **[53]**.

5.2 Pharmacokinetic analysis

PK parameters were calculated based on FVII:C, FVII:Ag, FX:C and FX:Ag levels. As shown in **Figs. 9A-D,** those levels rapidly increased after administration of MC710. FVII:C and FVII:Ag levels returned to pre-administration values during 12 to 24 h after the administration, and increased levels of FX:C and FX:Ag persisted in the blood until 48 h after the administration of MC710 at 80 μg kg^{-1} or more. The mean $t_{1/2}$ of FVII:C and FVII:Ag in the MC710-infused group was 2.1~3.4 h and 3.5~4.9 h, respectively, and that of FX:C and FX:Ag was 20.2~23.2 h and 22.8~27.5 h, respectively, shorter than reported values ($t_{1/2}$ of FX:C 24~56 h **[42, 43]**). On the other hand, the recovery of FVII:C and FVII:Ag in the MC710-infused group was 70.7~90.7% and 50.0~92.0%, respectively, and that of FX:C and FX:Ag was 98.7~120.9% and 94.0~109.4%, respectively. PK parameters of FVIIa were similar to previously reported values for rFVIIa **[41]**.

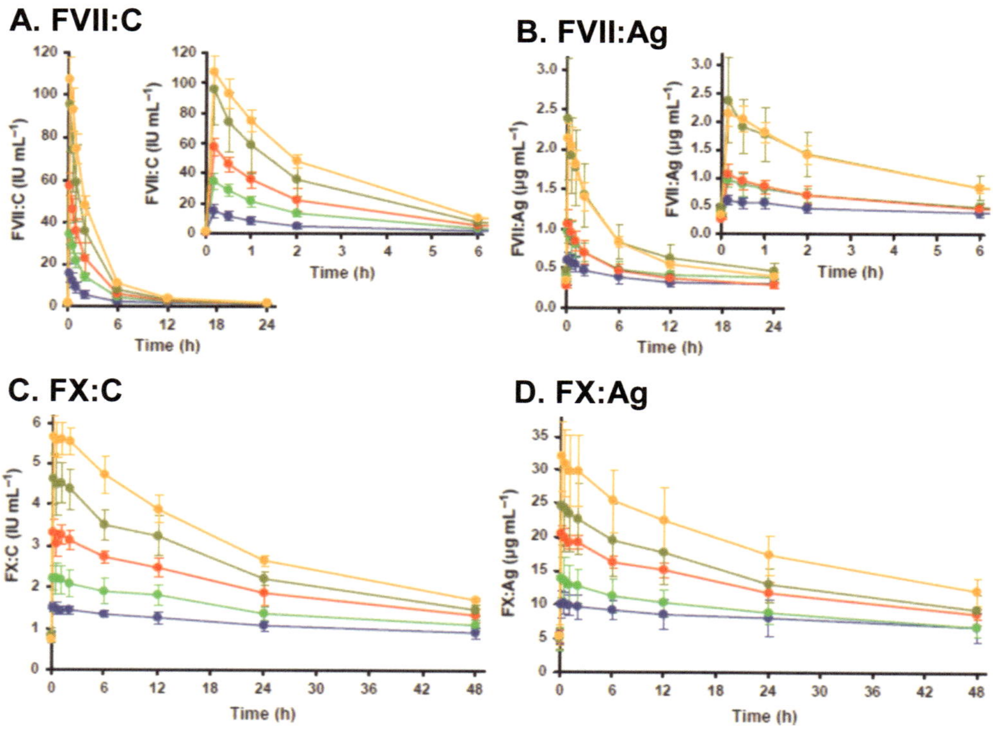

Time-dependent changes in the pharmacokinetics of FVII:C (Panel A), FVII:Ag (Panel B), FX:C (Panel C) and FX:Ag (Panel D) are shown. Enlarged figures of the changes in FVII:C and FVII:Ag until 6 hr after administration are shown in the right upper corner of each graph. The mark represents the mean ± SD. MC710 doses are denoted by the following color symbols: 20 μg kg^{-1}, (-●-); 40 μg kg^{-1}, (-●-); 80 μg kg^{-1}, (-●-); 100 μg kg^{-1}, (-●-); 120 μg kg^{-1}, (-●-). MC710 doses are denoted as FVIIa dose.

Fig. 9. Changes in pharmacokinetic parameters after the administration of MC710 to hemophilia patients with inhibitors(53)

5.3 Pharmacodynamic analysis

APTT and PT were measured as PD parameters. APTT, prolonged 120 sec or more before administration, improved in a dose-dependent manner after administration of MC710, and the effect persisted for 12 h at all doses **(Fig. 10A)**. At MC710 doses of more than 100 µg kg^{-1},

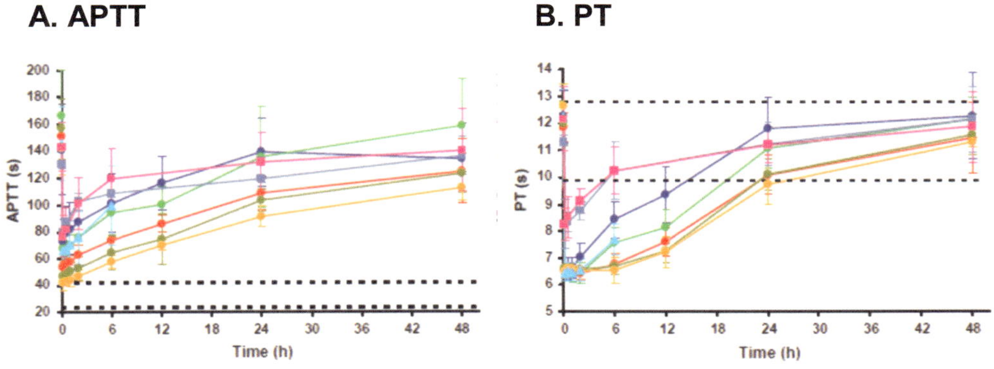

Time-dependent changes in APTT (Panel A) and PT (Panel B) are shown. The normal ranges for healthy individuals (- - -) for APTT were defined as 42.5 (upper limit) and 23.5 (lower limit) sec and for PT as 12.8 (upper limit) and 9.9 (lower limit) sec. The mark represents the mean ± SD. MC710, rFVIIa (NovoSeven®) and APCC (FEIBA®) doses are denoted by the following color symbols: MC710 (as FVIIa dose); 20 µg kg^{-1}, (-●-); 40 µg kg^{-1}, (-●-); 80 µg kg^{-1}, (-●-); 100 µg kg^{-1}, (-●-); 120 µg kg^{-1}, (-●-); rFVIIa; 120 µg kg^{-1}, (-▲-); APCC; 50 U kg^{-1}, (-■-); 75 U kg^{-1}, (-■-).

Fig. 10. Changes in pharmacodynamic parameters after the administration of MC710 to hemophilia patients with inhibitors(53)

the APTT was especially close to the normal range. Even 6 h after the administration of more than 100 µg kg^{-1} of MC710, the APTT was shorter than that immediately after the administration of 120 µg kg^{-1} of rFVIIa and 75 U kg^{-1} of APCC. It is expected that from the evaluation based on the level of improvement in APTT, the hemostatic effect immediately after the administration of MC710 at over 100 µg kg^{-1} might be equivalent to that of FVIII or FIX replacement therapy (replacement level 20 to 50% of these factors).

The PT reached approximately 6 sec (the determination limit) after administration of all doses of MC710 except for 20 µg kg^{-1} and remained at that level for up to 2 h. At 6 h after the administration of 80, 100 and 120 µg kg^{-1} of MC710, the PT was shorter than that after the administration of 120 µg kg^{-1} of rFVIIa. The reduction in PT persisted for 12 h at all doses **(Fig. 10B)**. The PT after the administration of 40, 80, 100 and 120 µg kg^{-1} of MC710 was shorter than that for 75 U kg^{-1} of APCC.

5.4 DIC and other safety concerns

TAT and F1+2 were increased after the administration of MC710 indicating the activation of prothrombin in blood flow; however, similar increases were also observed after the administration of rFVIIa and APCC **[54, 55]**. No serious or severe adverse events were observed within 4 weeks after the administration of MC710 and no subject discontinued treatment due to an adverse event. Also, no clinical symptoms or changes in laboratory tests (platelet count, fibrinogen, D-dimer) indicating a hypercoagulable state such as DIC were detected **(data not shown).** In addition, the results of virologic and serologic tests confirmed

that no subject developed a new viral antigen or produced a new antibody after the administration of MC710.

6. Conclusion and future perspectives

In this review, we described the rationale for the combined use of FVIIa and FX, the manufacturing process of FVIIa/FX mixture, MC710, and the treatment's prospective efficacy and safety. We also outlined the results of a Phase I clinical study. In the study, PK and PD parameters changed in a dose-dependent manner after the administration of MC710 and the changes in the PD parameters (APTT and PT) were equal to or greater than those in rFVIIa and APCC. Furthermore, MC710 was safely administered at doses of up to 120 μg kg^{-1} and no serious or severe adverse events, including DIC, were observed.

It was recently reported that the combination of APCC and rFVIIa is safe and effective in the treatment of bleeding that is unresponsive to monotherapy **[56].** This report supports our hypothesis that the FVIIa/FX mixture, MC710, would be a more potent bypassing agent than clinically available bypassing agents. Phase II clinical studies in hemophilia patients with inhibitors who are hemorrhaging have been completed in Japan and MC710 is expected to be used as an alternative to APCC and rFVIIa in the near future.

7. References

[1] Wight J, Paisley S. The epidemiology of inhibitors in hemophilia A: a systematic review. *Hemophilia* 2003;9:418-435.

[2] DiMichele D. Inhibitor development in hemophilia B: an orphan disease in need of attention. *Br J Haematol* 2007;138:305-15.

[3] Treur MJ, McCracken F, Heeg B, Joshi AV, Botteman MF, De Charro F, Van Hout B. Efficacy of recombinant activated factor VII vs. activated prothrombin complex concentrate for patients suffering from hemophilia complicated with inhibitors: a Bayesian meta-regression. *Hemophilia* 2009;15:420-36.

[4] Astermark J, Donfield SM, DiMichele DM, Gringeri A, Gilbert SA, Waters J, Berntorp E; FENOC Study Group. A randomized comparison of bypassing agents in hemophilia complicated by an inhibitor: the APCC RFVIIa Comparative (FENOC) Study. *Blood* 2007;109:546-51.

[5] Key NS, Christie B, Henderson N, Nelsestuen GL. Possible synergy between recombinant factor VIIa and prothrombin complex concentrate in hemophilia therapy. *Thromb Haemost* 2002;88:60-5.

[6] Schneiderman J, Rubin E, Nugent DJ, Young G. Sequential therapy with activated prothrombin complex concentrates and recombinant FVIIa in patients with severe hemophilia and inhibitors: update of our previous experience. *Haemophilia* 2007;13:244-8.

[7] Economou M, Teli A, Tzantzaroudi A, Tsatra I, Zavitsanakis A, Athanassiou-Metaxa M. Sequential therapy with activated prothrombin complex concentrate (APCC) and recombinant factor VIIa in a patient with severe hemophilia A, inhibitor presence and refractory bleeding. *Haemophilia* 2008;14:390-1.

[8] Livnat T, Martinowitz U, Zivelin A, Seligsohn U. Effects of factor VIII inhibitor bypassing activity (APCC), recombinant factor VIIa or both on thrombin generation in normal and hemophilia A plasma. *Haemophilia* 2008;14:782-6.

[9] Møss J, Scharling B, Ezban M, Møller Sørensen T. Evaluation of the safety and pharmacokinetics of a fast-acting recombinant FVIIa analogue, NN1731, in healthy male subjects. *J Thromb Haemost* 2009;7:299-305.
[10] Stennicke HR, Ostergaard H, Bayer RJ, Kalo MS, Kinealy K, Holm PK, Sørensen BB, Zopf D, Bjørn SE. Generation and biochemical characterization of glycoPEGylated factor VIIa derivatives. *Thromb Haemost* 2008;100:920-8.
[11] Prasad S, Lillicrap D, Labelle A, Knappe S, Keller T, Burnett E, Powell S, Johnson KW. Efficacy and safety of a new-class hemostatic drug candidate, AV513, in dogs with hemophilia A. *Blood* 2008;111:672-9.
[12] Morrissey JH, Macik BG, Neuenschwander PF, Comp PC. Quantitation of activated factor VII levels in plasma using a tissue factor mutant selectively deficient in promoting factor VII activation. *Blood* 1993;81:734-44.
[13] Wildgoose P, Nemerson Y, Hansen LL, Nielsen FE, Glazer S, Hedner U. Measurement of basal levels of factor VIIa in hemophilia A and B patients. *Blood* 1992;80:25-8.
[14] Higashi S, Matsumoto N, Iwanaga S. Molecular mechanism of tissue factor-mediated acceleration of factor VIIa activity. *J Biol Chem* 1996;271:26569-74
[15] Davie EW, Fujikawa K, Kisiel W. The coagulation cascade: initiation, maintenance, and regulation. *Biochemistry* 1991;30:10363-70.
[16] Goto S, Salomon DR, Ikeda Y, Ruggeri ZM. Characterization of the unique mechanism mediating the shear-dependent binding of soluble von Willebrand factor to platelets. *J Biol Chem* 1995;270:23352-61.
[17] Moroi M, Jung SM, Nomura S, Sekiguchi S, Ordinas A, Diaz-Ricart M. Analysis of the involvement of the von Willebrand factor-glycoprotein Ib interaction in platelet adhesion to a collagen-coated surface under flow conditions. *Blood* 1997;90:4413-24.
[18] Tomokiyo K, Kamikubo Y, Hanada T, Araki T, Nakatomi Y, Ogata Y, Jung SM, Nakagaki T, Moroi M. Von Willebrand factor accelerates platelet adhesion and thrombus formation on a collagen surface in platelet-reduced blood under flow conditions. *Blood* 2005;105:1078-84.
[19] Kulkarni S, Dopheide SM, Yap CL, Ravanat C, Freund M, Mangin P, Heel KA, Street A, Harper IS, Lanza F, Jackson SP. A revised model of platelet aggregation. *J Clin Invest* 2000;105:783-91
[20] Hedner U: Recombinant activated factor VII as a universal haemostatic agent. *Blood Coagul Fibrinolysis* 1998;Suppl 1:147-52
[21] van 't Veer C, Golden NJ, Mann KG: Inhibition of thrombin generation by the zymogen factor VII: implications for the treatment of hemophilia A by factor VIIa. *Blood* 2000;95:1330-1335
[22] Butenas S, Brummel KE, Branda RF, Paradis SG, Mann KG. Mechanism of factor VIIa-dependent coagulation in hemophilia blood. *Blood* 2002;99:923-30
[23] Monroe DM, Hoffman M, Oliver JA, Roberts HR: Platelet activity of high-dose factor VIIa is independent of tissue factor. *Br J Haematol* 1997;99:542-47.
[24] Monroe DM, Hoffman M, Oliver JA, Roberts HR: A possible mechanism of action of activated factor VII independent of tissue factor. *Blood Coagul Fibrinolysis* 1998;Suppl 1:15-20
[25] Hoffman M, Monroe DM.The action of high-dose factor VIIa (FVIIa) in a cell-based model of hemostasis. *Semin Hematol* 2001;38(Suppl 12):6-9.
[26] Weeterings C, de Groot PG, Adelmeijer J, Lisman T. The glycoprotein Ib-IX-V complex contributes to tissue factor-independent thrombin generation by recombinant factor VIIa on the activated platelet surface. *Blood* 2008;112:3227-33.

[27] Kenet G, Lubetsky A, Luboshitz J, Martinowitz U. A new approach to treatment of bleeding episodes in young hemophilia patients: a single bolus mega dose of recombinant activated factor VII (rFVIIa). *J Thromb Haemost* 2003;1:450-5.

[28] Kavakli K, Makris M, Zulfikar B, Erhardtsen E, Abrams ZS, Kenet G; RFVIIa trial (F7HAEM-1510) investigators. Home treatment of haemarthroses using a single dose regimen of recombinant activated factor VII in patients with hemophilia and inhibitors. A multi-centre, randomised, double-blind, cross-over trial. *Thromb Haemost* 2006;95:600-5.

[29] Chen SW, Pellequer JL, Schved JF, Giansily-Blaizot M. Model of a ternary complex between activated factor VII, tissue factor and factor IX. *Thromb Haemost* 2002;88:74-82.

[30] Kittur FS, Manithody C, Rezaie AR. Role of the N-terminal epidermal growth factor-like domain of factor X/Xa. *J Biol Chem* 2004;279:24189-96.

[31] Ndonwi M, Broze G Jr, Bajaj SP. The first epidermal growth factor-like domains of factor Xa and factor IXa are important for the activation of the factor VII-tissue factor complex. *J Thromb Haemost* 2005;3:112-8.

[32] Komiyama Y, Pedersen AH, Kisiel W. Proteolytic activation of human factors IX and X by recombinant human factor VIIa: effects of calcium, phospholipide and tissue factors. *Biochemistry* 1990;29:9418-25.

[33] Turecek PL, Varadi K, Keil B, Negrier C, Berntorp E, Astermark J, Bordet JC, Morfini M, Linari S, Schwarz HP. Factor VIII inhibitor-bypassing agents act by inducing thrombin generation and can be monitored by a thrombin generation assay. *Pathophysiol Haemost Thromb* 2003;33:16-22

[34] Fair DS, Plow EF, Edgington TS. Combined functional and immunochemical analysis of normal and abnormal human factor X. *J Clin Invest* 1979;64:884-94.

[35] Hemker HC, Giesen PL, Ramjee M, Wagenvoord R, Beguin S. The thrombogram: monitoring thrombin generation in platelet-rich plasma. *Thromb Haemost* 2000;83:589-91.

[36] Castoldi E, Rosing J. Thrombin generation tests. *Thromb Res* 2011;127(Suppl 3):S21-5.

[37] Brummel-Ziedins KE, Vossen CY, Butenas S, Mann KG, Rosendaal FR. Thrombin generation profiles in deep venous thrombosis. *J Thromb Haemost* 2005 ;3:2497

[38] Váradi K, Negrier C, Berntorp E, Astermark J, Bordet JC, Morfini ML-1inari S, Schwarz HP, Turecek PL. Monitoring the bioavailability of APCC with a thrombin generation assay. *J Thromb Haemost* 2005;3:2497-505.

[39] Hemker HC, Al Dieri R, De Smedt E, Béguin S.Thrombin generation, a function test of the haemostatic-thrombotic system. *Thromb Haemost* 2006;96:553-61.

[40] Nakatomi Y, Nakashima T, Gokudan S, Miyazaki H, Tsuji M, Hanada-Dateki T, Araki T, Tomokiyo K, Hamamoto T, Ogata Y. Combining FVIIa and FX into a mixture which imparts a unique thrombin generation potential to hemophilic plasma: an in vitro assessment of FVIIaFX mixture as an alternative bypassing agent. *Thromb Res* 2010;125:457-63.

[41] Lindley CM, Sawyer WT, Macik BG, Lusher J, Harrison JF, Baird-Cox K, Birchlazer S, Roberts HR. Pharmacokinetics and pharmacodynamics of recombinant factor VIIa. *Clin Pharmacol Ther* 1994;55:638-48.

[42] Mori K, Sakai H, Nakano N, Suzuki S, Sugai K, Hisa S, Goto Y. Congenital factor X deficiency in Japan. *Tohoku J Exp Med* 1981;133:1-19.

[43] Ostermann H, Haertel S, Knaub S, Kalina U, Jung K, Pabinger I. Pharmacokinetics of Beriplex PN prothrombin complex concentrate in healthy volunteers. *Thromb Haemost* 2007;98:790-7.
[44] Tomokiyo K, Nakatomi Y, Araki T, Teshima K, Nakano H, Nakagaki T, Miyamoto S, Funatsu A, Iwanaga S. A novel therapeutic approach combining human plasma-derived factors VIIa and X for haemophiliacs with inhibitors: evidence of a higher thrombin generation rate in vitro and more sustained haemostatic activity *in vivo* than obtained with factor VIIa alone. *Vox Sang* 2003;85:290-9.
[45] Bjoern S, Thim L. Activation of coagulation factor VII to VIIa. *Research Disclosure* 1986;269:564-65.
[46] Tomokiyo K, Yano H, Imamura I, Nakano Y, Nakagaki T, Ogata Y, Terano T, Miyamoto S, Funatsu A. Large-scale production and properties of human plasma-derived activated factor VII concentrate. *Vox Sang* 2003;84:54-64.
[47] Downey C, Kazmi R, Toh CH. Early identification and prognostic implications in disseminated intravascular coagulation through transmittance waveform analysis. *Thromb Haemost* 1998;80:65-9.
[48] Matsumoto T, Wada H, Nishioka Y, Nishio M, Abe Y, Nishioka J, Kamikura Y, Sase T, Kaneko T, Houdijk WP, Nobori T, Shiku H. Frequency of abnormal biphasic aPTT clot waveforms in patients with underlying disorders associated with disseminated intravascular coagulation. *Clin Appl Thromb Hemost.* 2006;12:185-92
[49] Shima M. Understanding the hemostatic effects of recombinant factor VIIa by clot wave form analysis. *Semin Hematol.* 2004;41(Suppl 1):125-31.
[50] Fukui H, Fujimura Y, Takahashi Y, Mikami S, Yoshioka A: Laboratory evidence of DIC under FEIBA treatment of a hemophilic patient with intracranial bleeding and high titer factor VIII inhibitor. *Thromb Res* 1981;22:177-184
[51] Rodeghiero F, Castronovo S, Dini E: Disseminated intravascular coagulation after infusion of FEIBA (factor VIII inhibitor bypassing activity) in a patient with acquired hemophilia. *Thromb Haemost* 1982;48:339-40
[52] Chavin SI, Siegel DM, Rocco TA, Olson JP: Acute myocardial infarction during treatment with an activated prothrombin complex concentrate in a patient with factor VIII deficiency and a factor VIII inhibitor. *Am J Med* 1988;85:245-9
[53] Shirahata A, Fukutake K, Mimaya J, Takamatsu J, Shima M, Hanabusa H, Takedani H, Takashima Y, Matsushita T, Tawa A, Higasa S, Takata N, Sakai M, Kawakami K, Ohashi Y, Saito H. Clinical pharmacological study of a plasma-derived factor VIIa and factor X mixture (MC710) in haemophilia patients with inhibitors - Phase I trial. *Haemophilia* 2011 in press
[54] Shirahata A, Kamiya T, Takamatsu J, Kojima T, Fukutake K, Arai M, Hanabusa H, Tagami H, Yoshioka A, Shima M, Naka H, Fujita S, Minamoto Y, Kamizono J, Saito H. Clinical trial to investigate the pharmacokinetics, pharmacodynamics, safety, and efficacy of recombinant factor VIIa in Japanese patients with hemophilia with inhibitors. *Int J Hematol* 2001;73:517-25.
[55] Elg M, Carlsson S, Gustafsson D. Effect of activated prothrombin complex concentrate or recombinant factor VIIa on the bleeding time and thrombus formation during anticoagulation with a direct thrombin inhibitor. *Thromb Res* 2001;101:145-57.
[56] Gringeri A, Fischer K, Karafoulidou A, Klamroth R, López-Fernández MF, Mancuso E; ON BEHALF OF THE EUROPEAN HAEMOPHILIA TREATMENT STANDARDISATION BOARD (EHTSB). Sequential combined bypassing therapy is safe and effective in the treatment of unresponsive bleeding in adults and children with hemophilia and inhibitors. *Haemophilia* 2011 in press

7

Mixed Genotypes in Hepatitis C Virus Infection

Patricia Baré and Raúl Pérez Bianco
Instituto de Investigaciones Hematológicas
Academia Nacional de Medicina, Fundación de la Hemofilia
Argentina

1. Introduction

Before the existence of commercial clotting factor concentrates, bleeding was the number one cause of death in persons with hemophilia and the only alternative treatment was cryoprecipitate. During the 1970s human freeze-dried (lyophilized) FVIII and FIX became available. The life of individuals with hemophilia was revolutionized because patients were able to treat themselves conveniently at home, as soon as spontaneous bleeds occurred. The commercial blood-derived products had a tremendous positive impact on physical, psychological and social lives. Unfortunately, they also carried an increased risk of blood-borne viral infections, largely due to their preparation from pools of plasma collected from thousands of donors. Consequently, the use of clotting factor concentrates resulted in human immunodeficiency virus (HIV) and hepatitis C virus (HCV) epidemics in this population (Lee C, 1995, 2009; Eyster, 2008; Ragni et al., 2010).

As reported in different cohorts around the world, many patients with hemophilia became infected with HIV between 1982 and 1985. In some hemophilic populations, subsequent testing of stored frozen plasma samples revealed that the first infections with HIV occurred in 1978-79, that the bulk of patients were infected in 1981-82, and that there were very few new infections by the end of 1984 (Eyster, 2008; Goedert et al., 1985).

The HCV epidemic was a much longer one, occurring between 1961 and 1985. The first patients became infected from the first large pool plasma-derived FIX concentrates and the epidemic ended with the dry heating of concentrates in 1985 (Lee C, 2009).

Particularly in Argentina, commercial factor concentrates were not accessible until 1975. As a result of the economic situation of the country, the non-availability of more expensive products leaded to a lower rate of HIV-infected people that reached 17% of our hemophilic population. Heat-inactivated factor concentrates were not available until November 1985.

Virtually, all hemophiliacs who received clotting factor concentrates prior to implementation of viral inactivation techniques became infected with hepatitis C virus at the time of the first infusion (Morfini et al, 1994; Lee C et al, 2002; Ragni et al, 2010). Prevalence rates of HCV infection up to 100% were reported in hemophilia patients treated with concentrates before 1985 (Yee et al., 2000; Lee C, 2009; Manucci, 2008; Arnold et al., 2006). Even though the introduction of heat-treated factor concentrates progressively decreased HCV transmission, the true risk ended when new regulations in blood donor screening together with the implementation of second and third generation immunoassays for the detection of antibodies against HCV was introduced in 1991 in Europe, in 1992 in the US and 1993 in

Argentina (Morfini et al., 1994; Franchini et al., 2001; Lee and Dusheiko, 2002; Tagliaferri et al., 2010; Argentinean Ministry of Health resolution #1077, 1993). However, it is important to notice that clotting factor concentrates used for Argentinean hemophilic patient treatments were never manufactured in the country but brought from the US or Europe.
Nowadays, viral inactivation and recombinant technologies have effectively prevented transfusion-transmitted viral pathogens in hemophilia. Though, due to the past chronic infections that occurred before viral inactivation procedures, transmissible agents continue to affect hemophilic population and hepatitis C represents a leading cause of morbidity and mortality in patients with hemophilia (Plug et al., 2006; Ragni et al., 2010).

2. HCV mixed genotype infections in hemophilic patients

HCV genotypes in individuals with hemophilia originate from variants within the infected donations used to manufacture factor concentrates or cryoprecipitate. Their HCV genotypes reflect the geographic distribution of genotypes from the blood donor population where the commercial products were manufactured (Jarvis et al., 1995, 1996; Fujimura et al., 1996; Preston et al., 1995; Toyoda et al., 1998; Tuveri R et al., 1997). Studies conducted within different groups provided no evidence that HCV genotypes differ significantly from each other in replication rate, transmissibility, or infectivity. However, selective transmission of HCV isolates during experimental chimpanzee infections and among humans exposed to commercially prepared factor VIII concentrate (lot DO56) containing multiple HCV species has also been suggested (Nainan et al., 2006).
The analysis of genotype distribution showed that several HCV genotypes might be circulating simultaneously in adults with hemophilia who received clotting factor concentrates before 1985 (Jarvis et al., 1995; Eyster et al., 1999; Schröter et al., 2003). Genotyping studies of multitransfused haemophiliacs suggested that the frequency of HCV mixed infection is high in this group but dissimilar rates of mixed infections were reported by different groups (Table 1).
Possible explanations for mixed infections in this population include exposure to multiple viruses from receipt of clotting factor concentrates prepared from multiple donors but also, combined with the absence of protective immunity following initial exposure to the virus (Farci et al., 1992) , from exposure to multiple viruses over time among repeated infusions, prior to HCV testing and inactivation.
When individuals are infected with more than one genotype, changes in the predominant genotype over time could be observed. As a result of immunologic pressure, genetic interaction between virus and host, or treatment intervention, the establishment of the dominant genotype may change over time (Jarvis et al., 1995; Eyster et al., 1999; Schröter et al., 2003).
Genotype changes were noted more frequently in the HIV-positive subjects than in the HIV-negative subjects. Some reports provided evidence of association between HIV status and the likelihood of HCV genotype to change, possibly related to loss of immune function and a consequent greater susceptibility to the new predominant viral variant (Jarvis et al., 1995; Eyster et al., 1999).
In the hemophilic population, changes in HCV genotype could be due to reactivation or reinfection but depending on which period is being evaluated is more likely to find one or the other. If the genotype shift precedes the implementation of heat-inactivated concentrates (1985), it is not easy to attribute the genotype change to HCV reactivation or reinfection.

Though, if the change in predominant genotype occurs after 1991-1992, when the true risk of HCV transmission through blood products ended, it is more likely to be due to reactivation rather than reinfection, assuming the absence of other patient's risk factors.

Author	*Year*	*% HCV mixed infections*	*Number of patients*	*Country*
Jarvis LM et al	1994	31	29	UK
Isobe K et al	1995	31	63	Japan
Tagariello G et al	1995	11	36	Italy
Preston FE et al	1995	7	96	UK
Fujimura Y et al	1996	12	74	Japan
Takayama S et al	1997	46.7	80	Japan
Tuveri R et al	1997	4 (5'NC region)	45	France
		18 (core region)		
Toyoda H et al	1999	20.8	53	Japan
Eyster E et al	1999	6 (1985-87)	32	US
		3 (1988-95)		
Toyoda H et al	1998	22	63	Japan
Schroter M et al	2003	2.2	600	Germany
Buckton et al	2006	19	37	UK
Samini Rad et al	2007	27.6	34	Iran

Table 1. Rates of HCV mixed infections in haemophilia

Some groups investigated the dynamics of the change in genotype in more detail, analyzing series of samples from different time points. There was no obvious trend towards replacement with any particular variant (Jarvis et al., 1995; Eyster et al., 1999).
Regardless the origin of the genotype shift (reinfection or reactivation), it could be revealing the presence of a mixed infection in the hemophilic patient.

3. Complications in assessing HCV mixed-genotype infections

A well-recognized deficiency of most genotyping assays is their limited sensitivity for detecting HCV mixed-genotype infections. The rate of HCV mixed infections is extremely dissimilar in the same type of patients described by different scientific groups. As seen in Table 1, the reported prevalence is variable depending on the genotyping methodology used. The difficulties of assessing the true prevalence of mixed infections in patients with multiple exposures remain a matter of concern (Bowden et al., 2005).
Although the prevalence and the mechanisms of HCV compartmentalization are still unknown, the presence of different HCV viral variants and different genotypes in different

tissues or compartments has been observed and could be associated with the existence of extrahepatic replication sites. This fact might result in additional complications to the analysis of HCV genotype in hemophilic patients.

3.1 Methods for HCV genotyping and limitations with mixed infections

The currently available assays, including direct DNA sequencing are designed to identify only the HCV genotype dominant in the population. Most of these techniques share the requirement of an initial target amplification step to generate suitable amounts of template for genotypic analysis. The PCR-resulting sequence for genotypic analysis may be generated by the viral isolate with the highest concentration in the serum or the one that preferentially binds to the primers used for the PCR (polymerase chain reaction). As a result, genotypes present at lower proportional levels in a mix or with lower affinity could be missed or mistyped (Hnatyszyn, 2005).

Both direct sequencing and restriction fragment length polymorphism assays seem to require 10% to 30% prevalence of minor strains before they can detect them (Qian et al., 2000; Frederick, 2010).

Hybridization based genotyping methods represent an attractive genotyping option compared to sequencing methods. The potential advantage of hybridization assays is their ability to detect mixed populations of virus with a prevalence as low as 2% (Qian et al., 2000). However similar to most genotyping methods, it involves PCR amplification of target regions of the viral genome and is confined by the advantages and disadvantages associated with PCR (Hnatyszyn, 2006; Frederick, 2010). It was reported that the latest version of the LiPA (Versant LiPA v2.0, Bayer HealthCare–Diagnostics), which targets both the 5′ UTR and the core protein, seems to have improved on the problem of subtyping and has performed better than a direct sequencing assay (Trugene) as well as an earlier version of the hybridization assay (Versant LiPA v1.0). The addition of sequences from the core protein has allowed better distinction between subtypes 1a and 1b as well as subtypes c to l of genotype 6 (Bouchardeau et al., 2007).

Population-based DNA sequencing (i.e., cloning and sequencing of HCV cDNA) is so far, an accurate method for detection of mixed-genotype infections; however, this is not routinely feasible because it is time consuming and expensive. In addition, several clones would need to be completely sequenced in the presence of multiple coexisting genotypes (Frederick, 2010).

3.2 Different genotypes in different reservoirs

Compartmentalization between different tissues of the same patient (serum-brain, serum-saliva, serum-peripheral blood mononuclear cells) was described in several studies (Radkowski et al., 2002; Roque Afonso et al., 2005). Furthermore, the existence of different genotypes and/or viral variants in different tissues of the same patient has been also demonstrated (Radkowski et al., 2002; Roy et al., 1998) and particularly, peripheral blood mononuclear cells can harbor distinct HCV variants that are not detected in plasma samples (Di Liberto et al., 2006, Roque-Afonso et al, 2005); adding a potential complication to the assessment of the correct HCV genotype.

As a consequence of unknown and multiple host-viral factors, different HCV genotypes between compartments (liver and extrahepatic reservoirs) could be reflecting true different viral variant proportions. Alternatively, they could be the consequence of technical inabilities to detect minor components with the same efficiency in a mixed population.

4. Importance of HCV genotype analysis

Hepatitis C virus genotype has been described as an independent response predictor for antiviral therapy. Its analysis, in combination with viral load, serves to optimize the therapeutic regimen (Zeuzem et al., 2004). Considering the fact some genotypes could be more resistant than others (Hayashi et al., 2006), most treatment protocols require the correct identification of the infecting HCV genotype to provide the dose and duration of antiviral therapy.

Revealing the occult genotypes might be necessary to choose the adequate antiviral therapy because strains that are not detected could have an unexpected impact on treatment. Furthermore, recurrence from reservoirs has been suggested (de Felipe B et al., 2008; Lee WM, et al., 2005).

5. HCV mixed-genotype infections in a population with hemophilia – Experience in Argentina

Our studies rely in a group of individuals with hemophilia extensively evaluated who is assisted at the Fundación Argentina de la Hemofilia through clinical visits and periodic diagnostic studies.

Using a cell culture system that allows the detection of the HCV genome during prolonged time periods (Baré et al., 2005), we investigated the presence of HCV in peripheral blood mononuclear cell (PBMC) cultures and the HCV genotypes associated to the lymphoid cells. Although peripheral blood mononuclear cells (PBMC) are not the primary site of HCV replication, previous reports emphasize their role as viral reservoirs (Radkowski et al., 2005; Pham et al., 2004). Furthermore, different genotypes have been reported both in plasma and PBMC (Roque Afonso et al., 2005) and it has also been speculated that extrahepatic HCV diversity may be an important determinant of treatment response (Blackard et al., 2007).

The final purpose of our study was to investigate the existence of unapparent HCV mixed infections in the hemophilic population in Argentina, analyzing the HCV genotypes detected in plasma or serum samples and comparing them to viral strains emerging under long-term PBMC cultures.

5.1 Cell culture system – Methodology details

Patient's PBMC derived from EDTA anti-coagulated blood samples, obtained at different time points, were cultured following the culture methodology (Ruibal et al., 2001). Briefly, PBMC were obtained by Ficoll-Paque PLUS density gradient (GE Healthcare, Bio- Sciences, USA). Cells were washed three times with Dulbecco's phosphate buffered saline 10X (Sigma Aldrich, USA) (PBS) and suspended to one million cells per milliliter in RPMI 1640 tissue culture medium (Hyclone RPMI-1640 medium 1X, Hyclone laboratories, Utah, USA) containing 10% fetal bovine serum and antibiotics (penicillin/streptomycin, 10 mg/ml) (RPMI-FBS). Two million cells were suspended in 2 ml RPMI-FBS using round-bottom 5 ml polystyrene tubes and left undisturbed in a 5% CO_2 incubator. For each patient, 4 to 10 different tubes were set up. Beginning on day 5 - 6 of culture, half of the supernatant (SN) was replaced twice a week with fresh medium by gentle aspiration, avoiding cell pellet disturbance. The SNs collected were frozen for future studies.

From our previous experience, using non-stimulated prolonged PBMC culture as described here, the virus was released spontaneously from the in vivo infected cells and increased the

chance of finding minor HCV genotypes not detected in the bulk of PBMCs at day 0 (before culturing the cells) (data not shown).

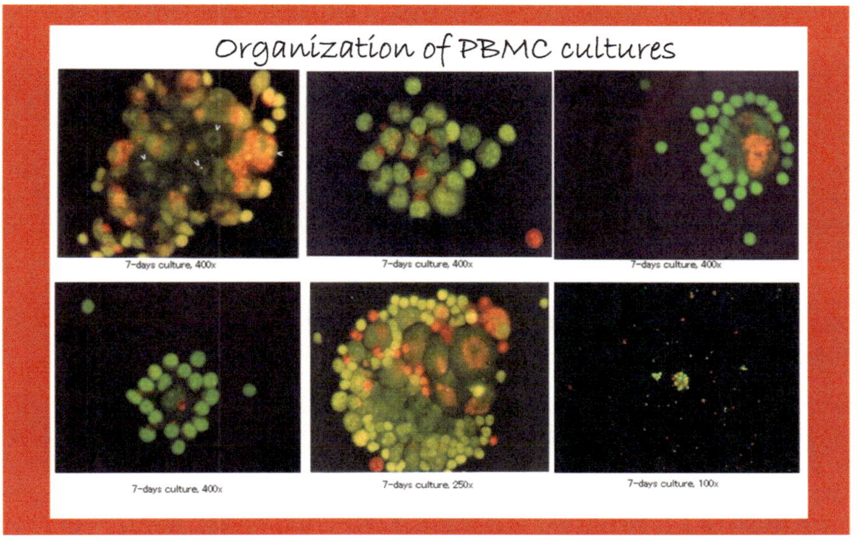

Fig. 1. Cell culture methodology (Ruibal et al.,1997): Organization of peripheral blood mononuclear cell cultures (PBMC). Aggregation of monocytes and lymphocytes is observed soon after the culture is started. Clumps containing T and B lymphocytes, dendritic cells and monocyte/macrophages are formed. Throughout the days, cell aggregates increase their size; monocyte/macrophages proliferate in close contact with lymphocytes and fuse into giant multinucleated cells. Apoptotic cells and debris are removed by activated macrophages.

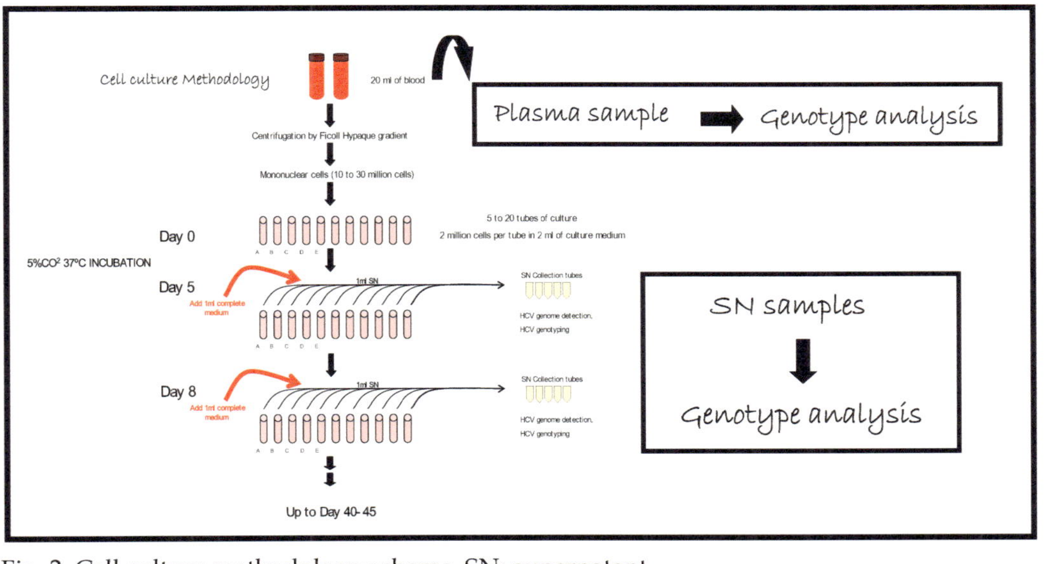

Fig. 2. Cell culture methodology scheme. SN: supernatant

5.2 HCV+ results in supernatants during cell culture

In our first report that was carried out studying only one culture per patient, HCV+ results were observed in 12 of 21 (57%) patients for the HCV monoinfected group and 23 of 31 (74%) of the coinfected group had HCV positive cultures (Baré et al., 2005). The difference between the populations did not reach statistical differences. However, in our longitudinally study involving 50 patients (25 HCV monoinfected and 25 HIV/HCV coinfected) and after analyzing 2 or 3 cell cultures per patient throughout 10 years of infection, almost every patient demonstrated at least one HCV+ PBMC culture. All of the HIV/HCV coinfected patients (25 of 25) and 92% (23 of 25) of the monoinfected individuals had HCV+ PBMC cultures.
During different weeks of culture, the rate of HCV+ SN for both groups was similar reaching 50 to 70 % during the first week. As the culture progressed, the percentage of HCV+ results in monoinfected population decreased gradually and generally, disappeared after the 4th week. Conversely, in the coinfected population HCV positivity remained longer.

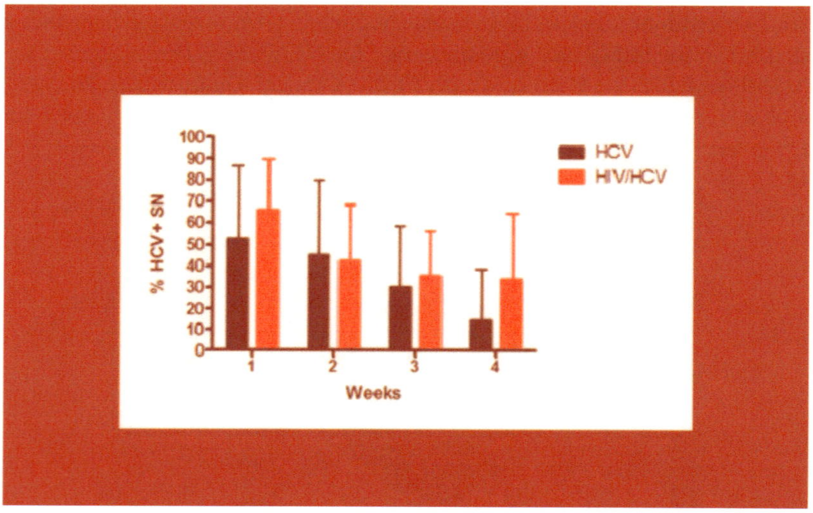

Fig. 3. HCV positivity in culture supernatants. Detection of HCV genome in cell culture supernatants during 4 weeks of culture. The percentage of HCV+ cell cultures for HIV/HCV coinfected and HCV monoinfected group were similar. HCV positivity decreased along the days of culture in both groups.

HCV recovery in supernatants appeared intermittently along the days of culture. HCV+ PCR results alternated with HCV negative results. The rate of HCV genome recovery in cell-free supernatant was used as an estimation of viral burden in the cells. Frequencies of HCV+ results out of the total SNs were analyzed.

$$\% \text{ HCV+} = \frac{\text{number of HCV RNA+ SNs} \times 100}{\text{total number of SN examined}}$$

The percentage of HCV+ SN in cell culture from the whole population ranged from 3 to 79% with a median value of 41.4% and a mean of 38.6%. The analysis of HCV+ percentages in different cultures from the same individual demonstrated that HCV positivity remained stable when considering only cultures from patients without HCV treatment.

The HCV genome was present at very low level with a mean value for coinfected patients of 3.39 ± 0.34 log (IU/ml) and 3.37± 0.26 log (IU/ml) for the HCV group (as reported in our first study). That could be the reason for the observed intermittent signal in the PCR results. Although there were no statistical differences between populations, the duration of the positive signal for more than 4 weeks in the coinfected group was remarkable.
Trying to find any clinical or viral related factor to the chance of originating an HCV+ culture, we found that the frequency of HCV+ results did not correlate with HCV or HIV viremia, neither HCV nor HIV viral loads in plasma samples. However, the patients with CD4+ counts lower than 250 cells/mm^3 were associated to higher frequencies of HCV+ results in cell cultures. It could be postulated that the low CD4+ cell counts that is a consequence of HIV infection could be related to a deficient control of HCV in culture.

5.3 HCV genotypes in plasma samples and culture supernatants

HCV genotype distribution was assessed in a group of 288 HCV chronically infected patients with hemophilia. Most of them were evaluated with one single plasma sample. All patients included in the study had a positive test for HCV antibodies detected by EIA assay (3rd generation) and RIBA 2.0 or 3.0 (both Ortho Clinical Diagnostics, Raritan, NJ, USA). Plasma samples were analyzed through genotyping techniques currently used for diagnosis (restriction fragment length polymorphisms and/or LIPA techniques).

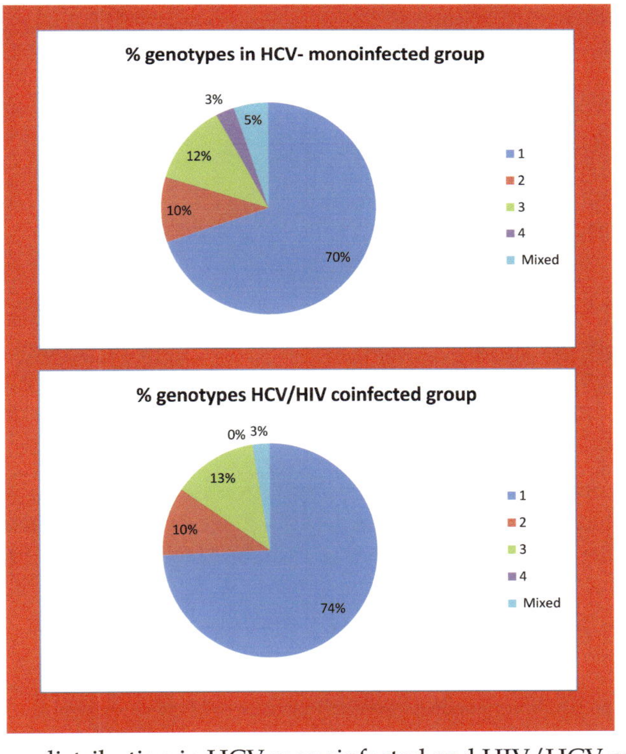

Fig. 4. HCV genotype distribution in HCV monoinfected and HIV/HCV coinfected group

The distribution of HCV genotypes in the hemophilic population in Argentina reflects the plasma donors in Europe and United States and was reported previously by Picchio et al, in 59

individuals, finding that HCV genotype 1 was the predominant viral variant detected among HIV-negative (76%) and HIV-positive (82.5%) patients, followed by genotypes 3 (10.4%), 2 (2%) and a small proportion of multiply co-infected patients including genotypes 4 and 5 (6.25%). In the group of 288 individuals, the HCV genotype distribution for the entire population was 72 % of genotype 1, 10% of genotype 2, 12% genotype 3 and 2.5 % of genotype 4. Similar distribution was observed when considering HCV mono-infected or HIV/HCV co-infected population (p>0.05). Taking into account different HCV genotypes (and not HCV subtypes) as shown in fig 4, mixed-genotype infections were observed in 5.6 % of the patients (Parodi et al., 2008).

Analysis of HCV genotypes associated to lymphoid cells found along cultures have previously demonstrated the presence of occult HCV mixed-genotype infections in 62% of 16 patients with hemophilia (Parodi et al., 2008).

In the present study, plasma and cell culture samples were longitudinally analyzed in 25 HCV monoinfected and 25 HIV/HCV coinfected individuals in a period of time between 1993 and 2010. Different time point cultures were evaluated. HCV genome presence and genotyping were analyzed as described previously (Parodi et al., 2008) on an average of 15 culture supernatants per time point. Plasma samples were also studied at different dates along the time period and for at least 3 time points for each individual. Genotypes found in plasma samples were compared to the correspondent samples obtained under culture.

Analyzing 3 or more sequential plasma samples included in the studied period, the 69% (33 of 48) of the patients showed genotype 1, 4% genotype 2 and 4% genotype 3 (2 of 48), 2% (1 of 48) genotype 4, while 21% (10 of 48) had mixed-genotyped HCV infections. Results in culture samples performed during the same time period showed the presence of genotype 1 in 46% (21 of 46) of the patients and mixed infections in 50% (23 of 46) of the subjects. The remaining 4% (2 of 46) was genotype 2. Using the cell culture system the chance of discovering mixed-HCV genotype infections was 3.8 times greater than with longitudinal analysis of plasma samples (OR=3.8, p= 0.005, 95%CI =1.54 - 9.4). However, also the analysis of serial plasma samples instead of one single plasma sample increased the chance of discovering mixed infections in 5.2 times (OR=5.2, p= 0.0006, 95%CI =2.15 – 12.5).

ID	Serial plasma samples	n	Genotypes in culture SN	n cult	nSN
HIV/HCV coinfected group					
1	1+2	10	1+2	3	44
2	1	9	1+2	3	40
3	1	8	1+2	3	62
4	1+2	9	1+2	4	59
5	1+2+3	9	1+3	4	119
6	1	9	1+3	6	101
7	1	7	1+2+3	3	45
8	1+4	9	1+4	4	61
14	1	6	1	4	63
15	1	8	1+2+3	4	53
16	1	6	1	3	34
17	1	5	1	4	52
26	1+3	7	1+2	3	42
27	1+3	6	1+2	4	63
29	1	6	1+2	3	41
30	2	6	2	3	48
35	1+3	4	1+3	3	41
39	1	5	1	2	28
40	1	4	1+3	3	45
41	1	3	1	2	32
42	1	3	1+3	2	29
43	1	5	1	2	32
47	-	5	1	2	32
48	3	3	1+3	2	48
49	-	5	2	2	32

ID	Serial plasma samples	n	Genotypes in culture SN	n cult	nSN
HCV monoinfected group					
9	4	3	1+2+3+4	2	54
10	1	7	1+2+3	2	34
11	1	5	1+2	2	38
12	1+3	6	1+3	3	44
13	1	4	1	3	29
18	1	4	1	2	26
19	1	3	1	2	22
20	1	3	1	2	9
21	1	4	1	2	24
22	1	5	1	2	29
23	1	4	1	3	40
24	1	5	1+3	2	28
25	1	3	1+2	2	29
28	1	3	1	1	14
31	3	8	-	2	30
32	1	4	1	2	29
33	1+2	4	-	2	22
34	1+3	6	-	2	30
36	1	3	1	2	31
37	1	4	1	2	29
38	1	4	1	2	21
44	2	5	1+2	2	32
45	1	6	-	2	31
46	1	3	1	1	15
50	1	5	1	1	16

Table 2. Genotypes in plasma and culture supernatants in 50 patients. SN: supernatant

From 23 subjects with HCV+ typeable supernatants in cell culture who showed mixed HCV genotypes, 16 were HIV/HCV coinfected and 7 HCV monoinfected patients. HIV infection was found to be associated to the possibility of having mixed genotype infection ($p=0.02$, $OR=4.57$, 95%CI =1.38 - 15.11).

6. Conclusion

In our experiments, distinct HCV genotypes associated to PBMC and not present in serial plasma samples were verified. Therefore, mononuclear cells might be acting as an independent viral reservoir in this cohort whether or not HCV replicates inside these cells.
Mononuclear cells might be involved in HCV persistence as an extrahepatic reservoir in this cohort. Even if HCV replication or cell adsorption were not explored in our experiments, the fact that we detected PBMC-associated genotypes throughout a long-time period is compatible with the existence of an extra-hepatic replication site. Otherwise, if extremely low or occult replication of lymphotropic variants was taking place in the liver, viral particles could be adsorbed preferentially to blood monocytes that continuously circulate through this tissue, and be detected thereafter in the PBMC cultures.
Techniques that involve cell culture and cloning methodologies are time-consuming, expensive and difficult to perform in a diagnostic facility. However, through the use of a reliable genotyping technique in combination with the analysis of multiple time points in an extended period of time, the chance to identify most of the infecting HCV genotypes, when mixed infections are present, could be increased.
The final goal of detecting the predominant together with minor HCV genotypes is to help to provide the proper dose and duration of antiviral therapy. Otherwise, changes in the predominant variant could have unexpected impact on the treatment response. The clinical and therapeutic implications of lymphotropic HCV variants related to their persistence requires further investigation, especially in hemophilic HIV/HCV coinfected persons.

7. Acknowledgements

The authors gratefully acknowledge Dr María Marta E de Bracco and Dr Miguel de Tezanos Pinto for helpful advice and the invaluable assistance of the staff of Virology and Immunology laboratories from Academia Nacional de Medicina: Natalia Aloisi, Mariela Bastón and Cecilia Monzani.
This study was supported by Bayer Haemophilia Awards Program (Bayer Healthcare), grants from SECYT PICT 0393-2008 and Fundación René Barón.
We are indebted to Fundación Argentina de la Hemofilia (health professionals, administrative staff and technicians) and the patients with hemophilia for their constant support and generous cooperation.

8. References

Alter, M.J.; Kruszon-Moran D.; Nainan, O.V.; McQuillan, G.M.; Gao, F.; Moyer, L.A.; Kaslow, R.A. & Margolis HS. (1999). The prevalence of hepatitis C virus infection in the United States, 1988 through 1994. *N Engl J Med*, 341, 556–562.

Arnold, D.M.; Julian, J.A. & Walker, I.R. (2006). Mortality rates and causes of death among all HIV-positive individuals with hemophilia in Canada over 21 years of follow-up. *Blood*. 108:460-4.

Baré, P. ; Massud, I. ; Parodi, C. ; Belmonte, L.; García, G.; Nebel, M.C.; Corti, M.; de Tezanos Pinto, M.; Pérez Bianco, R.; de Bracco, M.M.; Campos, R. & Ruibal Ares, B. (2005). Continuous release of Hepatitis C virus by peripheral blood mononuclear cells and B- lymphoblastoid cell line cultures, derived from HCV infected patients. *J Gen Virol*. 86: 1717-1727

Buckton, A.J.; Ngui,S.L.; Arnold, C.; Boast, K.; Kovacs, J.; Klapper, P.E.; Bharat Patel, B.; Ibrahim, I. ; Rangarajan, S.; Ramsay, M.E. & Teo, C.G. (2006). Multitypic Hepatitis C Virus Infection Identified by Real-Time Nucleotide Sequencing of Minority Genotypes. *J Clin Microbiol*. 44: 2779–2784

Blackard, J.T.; Hiasa, Y.; Smeaton, L.; Jamieson, D.J.; Rodriguez, I.; Mayer K.H. & Chung, R.T. (2007). Compartmentalization of hepatitis C virus (HCV) during HCV/HIV coinfection. *J Infect Dis*. 195: 1765-73.

Bouchardeau, F, ; Cantaloube, J.F. ; Chevaliez, S. ; Portal, C. ; Razer, A. ; Lefrère, J.J. ; Pawlotsky, J.M. ; De Micco, P. & Laperche S. (2007). Improvement of Hepatitis C Virus (HCV) Genotype Determination with the New Version of the INNO-LiPA HCV Assay. *J Clin Microbiol*. 45: 1140–1145

Bowden, S.; McCaw, R.; White, P.A.; Crofts, N. & Aitken CK. (2005). Detection of multiple hepatitis C virus genotypes in a cohort of injecting drug users. *J Viral Hepat*. 12: 322-324

de Felipe, B.; Leal, M.; Soriano-Sarabia, N.; Gutiérrez, A.; López-Cortés, L.; Molina-Pinelo, S. & Vallejo A. (2008). HCV RNA in peripheral blood cell subsets in HCV-HIV coinfected patients at the end of PegIFN/RBV treatment is associated with virologic relapse. *J Viral Hepat*. 16: 21-27

Di Liberto, G.; Roque-Afonso, A.M.; Kara, R.; Ducoulombier, D.; Fallot, G.; Samuel, D. & Féray, C. (2006) Clinical and therapeutic implications of hepatitis C virus compartmentalization. *Gastroenterology*. 131: 76-84.

Eyster, E. (2008). Coping with the HIV epidemic 1982–2007: 25-year outcomes of the Hershey Haemophilia Cohort. *Haemophilia*. 14:697–702

Eyster, M.E.; Sherman, K.E.; Goedert, J.J.; Katsoulidou, A. & Hatzakis, A. (1999). Prevalence and changes in hepatitis C virus genotypes among multitransfused persons with hemophilia. The Multicenter Hemophilia Cohort Study. *J Infect Dis*. 179(5):1062-9.

Farci, P.; Alter, H.J.; Govindarajan, S.; Wong, D.C.; Engle, R.; Lesniewski, R.R.; Mushahwar, I.K.; Desai, S.M.; Miller, R.H.; Ogata, N. & Purcell, R.H. (1992). Lack of protective immunity against reinfection with hepatitis C virus. *Science*. 258:135-140

Franchini, M.; Rossetti, G.; Tagliaferri, A.; Capra, F.; de Maria, E.; Pattacini, C.; Lippi, G.; Lo Cascio, G.; de Gironcoli, M. & Gandini, G. (2001). The natural history of chronic hepatitis C in a cohort of HIV-negative Italian patients with hereditary bleeding disorders. *Blood*. 98:1836-1841.

Frederick, R.T. (2010). Hepatitis C Assays: The Pitfalls of Polymerase Chain Reaction and Genotyping. *Curr Hepatitis Rep* 9:9–14

Fujimura, Y.; Ishimoto, S.; Shimoyama, T.; Narita, N.; Kuze, Y.; Yoshioka, A.; Fukui, H.; Tanaka, T.; Tsuda, F.; Okamoto, H.; Miyakawa, Y. & Mayumi, M. (1996). Genotypes

and multiple infections with hepatitis C virus in patients with haemophilia A in Japan. *J. Viral Hepatitis.* 3: 79-84.

Goedert, J.J.; Biggar, R.J.; Weiss, S.H.; Eyster, M.E.; Melbye, M.; Wilson, S.; Ginzburg, H.M.; Grossman, R.J.; DiGioia, R.A.; Sanchez, W.C.; Giron, J. A.; Ebbesen, P.; Gallo, R. C. & Blattner, W. A. (1985). Three-year incidence of AIDS in five cohorts of HTLV-III-infected risk group members. *Science.* 231: 992–5.

Hayashi, N. & Takehara, T. (2006). Antiviral therapy for chronic hepatitis C: past, present, and future. *J Gastroenterol.* 41:17-27.

Hnatyszyn, H.J. (2005). Chronic hepatitis C and genotyping: the clinical significance of determining HCV genotypes. *Antivir Ther.* 10: 1-11

Isobe, K.; Imoto, M.; Fukuda, Y.; Koyama, Y.; Nakano, I. ; Hayakawa, T. & Takamatsu, J. (1995). Hepatitis C virus infection and genotypes in Japanese hemophiliacs. *Liver.* 15:131-134.

Jarvis, L.M.; Ludlam, A.; & Simmonds P. (1995). Hepatitis C virus genotypes in multi-transfused individuals. *Haemophilia.* 1: 3-7

Jarvis, L.M.; Ludlam, C.A.; Ellender, J.A.; Nemes, L.; Field, S.P.; Song, E.; Chuansumrit, A.; Preston, F.E. & Simmonds, P. (1996). Investigation of the relative infectivity and pathogenicity of different hepatitis C virus genotypes in hemophiliacs. *Blood.* 87:3007–11.

Jarvis, L.M.; Watson, H.G.; McOmish, F.; Peutherer, J.F. ; Ludlam, C.A. & Simmonds P. (1994). Frequent reinfection and reactivation of hepatitis C virus genotypes in multitransfused hemophiliacs. *J Infect Dis.* 170:1018-22.

Lee, C. & Dusheiko, G. (2002). The natural history and antiviral treatment of hepatitis C in haemophilia. *Haemophilia.* 8:322-9.

Lee, C. (2009). The best of times, the worst of times: a story of haemophilia. *Clinical Medicine.* 9: 453–8

Lee, W.M.; Polson, J.E.; Carney, D.S.; Sahin, B. & Gale, M. Jr. (2005). Reemergence of hepatitis C virus after 8.5 years in a patient with hypogammaglobulinemia: evidence for an occult viral reservoir. *J Infect Dis.* 192: 1088-1092.

Mannucci, P. (2008). Back to the future: a recent history of haemophilia treatment. Haemophilia. 14: 10–18

Morfini, M. ; Mannucci, P.M.; Ciavarella, N.; Schiavoni, M.; Gringeri, A.; Rafanelli, D.; Di Bona, E.; Chistolini, A.; Tagliaferri, A.; Rodorigo, G.; Baudo, F. & Gamba, G. (1994). Prevalence of infection with the hepatitis C virus among Italian hemophiliacs before and after the introduction of virally inactivated clotting factor concentrates: a retrospective evaluation. *Vox Sang.* 67:178-82.

Nainan, O.V.; Lu, L.; Gao, F.X.; Meeks, E.; Robertson, B.H. & Margolis, H.S. (2006). Selective transmission of hepatitis C virus genotypes and quasispecies in humans and experimentally infected chimpanzees. *J Gen Virol.* 87: 83-91.

Parodi, C.; Culasso, A.; Aloisi, N.; García, G.; Bastón, M.; Corti, M.; Pérez Bianco, R.; Campos, R. ; Ruibal Ares, B. & Baré, P. (2008). Evidence of occult HCV genotypes in haemophilic individuals with unapparent HCV mixed infections. *Haemophilia.* 14: 816-822.

Pham, T.N.; MacParland, S.A.; Mulrooney, P.M.; Cooksley, H.; Naoumov, N.V. & Michalak, T.I. (2004). Hepatitis C virus persistence after spontaneous or treatment-induced resolution of hepatitis C. *J Virol.* 78: 5867-5874.

Picchio, G.R.; Nakatsuno, M.; Boggiano, C.; Sabbe, R.; Corti, M.; Daruich, J.; Pérez-Bianco, R.; Tezanos-Pinto, M.; Kokka, R.; Wilber, J. & Mosier, D. (1997). Hepatitis C (HCV) genotype and viral titer distribution among Argentinean hemophilic patients in the presence or absence of human immunodeficiency virus (HIV) co-infection. *J Med Virol*. 52: 219-225.

Plug, I.; Van Der Bom, J.G.; Peters, M.; Mauser-Bunschoten, E.P.; De Goede-Bolder, A. ; Heijnen, L.; Smit, C.; Willemse, J. & Rosendaal, F.R. (2006). Mortality and causes of death in patients with hemophilia, 1992-2001: a prospective cohort study. *J Thromb Haemost*. 4:510-6.

Preston, F. E.; Jarvis, L. M. ; Makris, M. ; Philp, L. ; Underwood, J. C. E. ; Ludlam, C. A. & Simmonds, P. (1995). Heterogeneity of hepatitis C virus genotypes in hemophilia and relationship with chronic liver disease. *Blood*. 85:1259-1262.

Qian, K.P.; Natov, S.N.; Pereira, B. J.G. & Lau, J.Y.N. (2000). Hepatitis C virus mixed genotype infection in patients on haemodialysis. *J. Viral Hepatitis*. 7, 153-160

Radkowski, M.; Gallegos-Orozco, J.F. ; Jablonska, J.; Colby, T.V.; Walewska-Zielecka, B.; Kubicka, J.; Wilkinson, J.; Adair, D.; Rakela, J. & Laskus, T. (2005). Persistence of hepatitis C virus in patients successfully treated for chronic hepatitis C. *Hepatology*. 41: 106-114.

Radkowski, M.; Wilkinson, J. ; Nowicki, M. ; Adair, D. ; Vargas, H. ; Ingui, C. ; Rakela, J. ; & Laskus, T. (2002). Search for hepatitis C virus negative-strand RNA sequences and analysis of viral sequences in the central nervous system: evidence of replication. *J Virol*. 76:600-608.

Ragni, M.V.; Sherman, K.E. & Jordan, J.A. (2010). Viral pathogens. *Haemophilia*. 5:40-6.

Roque-Afonso, A.M.; Ducoulombier, D.; Di Liberto, G.; Kara, R.; Gigou, M.; E. Dussaix, E.; Samuel, D. & Féray, C. (2005). Compartmentalization of hepatitis C virus genotypes between plasma and peripheral blood mononuclear cells. *J Virol*. 79:6349-6357.

Roy, K. M.; Bagg, J.; McCarron, B.; Good, T.; Cameron, S. & Pithie, A. (1998). Predominance of HCV type 2a in saliva from intravenous drug users. *J Med Virol*. 54:271–275.

Ruibal-Ares, B.; Riera, N.E. & Bracco, M.M.E. (1997). Macrophages, multinucleated giant cells, and apoptosis in HIV+ patients and normal blood donors. *Clin Immunol Immunopathol*. 82, 102–116.

Samini, R. & Shahbaz, B. (2007). Hepatitis C virus genotypes among patients with thalassemia and inherited bleeding disorders in Markazi province, Iran. *Haemophilia*. 13, 156–163

Schröter, M.; Heinz-Hubert, F.; Zöllner, B.; Schäfer, P. & Laufs, R. (2003). Multiple infections with different HCV genotypes: prevalence and clinical impact. *J Clin Virol*. 27: 200-204.

Tagariello, G. ; Pontisso, P. ; Davoli, P.G. ; Ruvoletto, M.G. ; Traldi, A. & Alberti A. (1995). Hepatitis C virus genotypes and severity of chronic liver disease in haemophiliacs. *Br J Haematol*. 91:708-13.

Tagliaferri, A.; Rivolta, G.F.; Iorio, A.; Oliovecchio, E. ; Mancuso, M.E.; Morfini, M.; Rocino, A.; Mazzucconi, M.G. & Franchini, M. (2010). Italian Association of Hemophilia Centers. Mortality and causes of death in Italian persons with haemophilia, 1990-2007. *Haemophilia*. 16:437-46.

Takayama, S.; Taki, M. ; Meguro, T. ; Nishikawa, K. ; Shiraki, K. & Yamada, K. (1997). Virological characteristics of HCV infection in Japanese haemophiliacs. *Haemophilia*. 3: 131-136

Todd, F. (2010). Hepatitis C Assays: The Pitfalls of Polymerase Chain Reaction and Genotyping R. *Curr Hepatitis Rep*. 9:9-14.

Toyoda, H.; Fukuda, Y.; Hayakawa, T.; Takayama, T.;Kumada, T.; Nakano, S.; Takamatsu, J. & Saito H. (1998). Characteristics of patients with chronic infection due to hepatitis C virus of mixed subtypes: Prevalence, viral RNA, and response to interferon therapy. *Clin Infect Dis*. 26: 440-445.

Tuveri, R.; Rothschild, C.; Pol, S. ; Reijasse, D.; Persico, T.; Gazengel, C.; Bréchot, C. & Thiers V. (1997). Hepatitis C virus genotypes in French haemophiliacs: kinetics and reappraisal of mixed infections. *J Med Virol*. 51(1):36-41.

Yee, T.T.; Griffioen, A.; Sabin, C.A.; Dusheiko, G. & Lee, C.A. (2000). The natural history of HCV in a cohort of haemophilic patients infected between 1961 and 1985. *Gut*. 47:845-51.

Zeuzem, S.; Hultcrantz, R.; Bourliere, M.; Goeser, T.; Marcellin, P.; Sanchez-Tapias, J.; Sarrazin, C.; Harvey, J.; Brass, C. & Albrecht, J. (2004). Peginterferon alfa-2b plus ribavirin for treatment of chronic hepatitis C in previously untreated patients infected with HCV genotypes 2 or 3. *J Hepatol*. 40(6):993-9.

8

Characteristics of Older Patient with Haemophilia

Silva Zupančić Šalek, Ana Boban and Dražen Pulanić
National Referral Haemophilia and Thrombophilia Centre, Division of Haematology
Department of Internal Medicine, University Hospital Centre Zagreb
Croatia

1. Introduction

The mankind is living longer due to improved quality of life, better healthcare service worldwide and less infant mortality. Progressive demographic ageing of the older population is a global process. The 80 or over age group is growing faster than any young segment of the older population

1.1 Life expectancy in patients with haemophilia

Until 1960 haemophilia was a life-threatening disease with limited treatment options as splints, icepacks and bed rest. With the discovery of factor concentrates the life of haemophilia patients changed dramatically better. They improved quality of life and prolong life expectancy (Mejia-Carvajal, 2006). Median life expectancy in males with severe haemophilia was 11 years in the early 20th century, increased to the range of 55 to 63 years in the 1970s (Plug, 2006; Darby, 2007). By the early 1980s life expectancy was almost 68 years (Chorba, 2001; Oldenburg, 2009). By 1990s the life expectancy in US haemophiliacs dropped to 49 years because of HIV infections. The decline in HIV-related mortality in HIV-infected persons with haemophilia reflected improvements in highly active anti-retroviral therapy (HAART). In 2001, haemophiliac life expectancy in The Netherlands reached 67 years (74 years for those without blood borne virus infections) and by 2007, the overall haemophilic life expectancy was reported to be 71 years in Italy (Plug, 2006; Tagliaferri, 2010) that is approaching the general male population. About 2% of haemophilia A and B patients surveyed in US comprehensive haemophilia treatment centres are 65 years of age or older and 15% are 45 years or older (Philipp, 2010).

1.2 Quality of life in patients with haemophilia

As haemophiliacs are reaching old age new problems are arising. Except physical problems we are faced today with psychological problems in older patients with haemophilia (Siboni, 2009). They are related to family dynamics (Franchini, 2007) and early retirement. Data on health-related quality of life (HR-QoL) of elderly persons with haemophilia are scare. Quality of life has become an important issue for physicians who are treating haemophilia patients and an increasing number of studies have analysed the HR-QoL in this population, using specific instruments for its measurement Haemo-QoL (Gringeri, 2006). Results from

multicentre study conducted in Italy in a cohort of elderly haemophiliacs (≥ 65 years) have shown similar cognitive status as elderly non-haemophiliacs. Persons with haemophilia report depression and lower health-related quality of life (Siboni, 2009). These results are very important because, the health status of elderly persons with haemophilia was evaluated in a case control study. These data are consistent with studies on HR-QoL in younger haemophilia patients (Scalone, 2006).

2. Characteristics of older haemophiliac

The life expectancy in persons with haemophilia is increasing and reaching almost that of e general population (Mejia-Carvajal, 2006). In many haemophilia centres, especially those in well-developed countries, old haemophilia person is not a rarity. Haematologists have little experience in managing the age related comorbidities of elderly haemophiliacs and the data are very rare. There is no evidence-based information to guide clinicians and help them to solve the problems. Population of haemophiliacs is aging slowly, giving us time to solve the problems and generate high quality data.

2.1 Haemophilia related comorbidities and age related diseases

Haemophilia patients with increased age suffer the same diseases as the normal male population, especially in well developed countries with sufficient quantity of factor concentrate (Franchini, 2009). Aging is bringing to haemophilia patients not only haemophilia related complications (arthropathy and chronic viral infections) or comorbidities but also age related diseases (cardiovascular disease, malignancy, renal disease, osteoporosis, mental diseases, etc.). About 88% of the general population over the age of 65 years have one or more chronic medical conditions (Hoffman, 1995). Today, clinical experience about comorbidities in elderly haemophiliacs and their influence on the primary disorder, haemophilia are lacking.

2.1.1 Arthropathy

Haemophilia A and B are characterized in the most severe form with spontaneous bleeding into joints and muscles. Prophylactic therapy with factor concentrates has been shown, if started early, reduce the burden of haemophilic arthropathy (Dolan, 2010; Kulkarni, 2003). Administration of factor concentrate on regular basis, prophylactically demonstrated in US Joint Outcome study benefits in preventing joint damage and bleeding episodes, compared with on-demand use in children (Manco-Johnson, 2007). It is known that many adults with severe haemophilia over the age of 65 and older did not have adequate access for regular treatment until adulthood. They have established haemophilic arthropathy with typical joint deformity, muscle weakness and impaired proprioception (Nilsson, 1992; Siboni, 2009) that influence the quality of life (limitations in their daily activities, etc.). Italian study was the first to evaluate the general health status in patients with severe haemophilia, aged ≥65 years and were compared with elderly men without bleeding disorders matched for age, sex, geography and social status. Almost all patients with haemophilia had arthropathy, except two. More than half were affected in all six joints considered (57%): only one patient was affected in one joint only, five in three joints and the remaining 28 patients in more than three joints. Haemophilia patients had higher pain score and significant difference was found in the orthopaedic score between the two groups. No statistical difference was found for the number of surgical procedures but joint arthroplasty was performed in 46% of

patients with haemophilia and 7% in non-haemophilic (Siboni, et al 2009). Orthopaedic surgical procedures are usually ankle arthrodesis, osteotomy, hip and knee arthroplasty. Indications for such procedures are chronic permanent pain in arthropathic joint, disability and ineffectiveness of conservative management. There will be more revision operations that have a higher risk of bleeding, in older haemophilia patients who had their first arthroplasty about 15 years earlier. Perioperative treatment for orthopaedic surgery is administration of factor concentrate to achieve normal activity of F VIII as well as protects from development of thromboembolism.

Two approaches are applying for thromboprophylaxis: administration of low molecular weight heparins shortly after operation and under the cover of factor concentrates or using mechanical methods with early ambulation. Thromboprophylaxis is still a big question with certain controversial. Proprioceptive loss seen in elderly haemophiliacs could increase the risk of falls (Street, 2006). About 70% of elderly people with haemophilia had a high risk of falling, spontaneously or after tripling on obstacles (Siboni, 2009). Physical therapy is essential part of comprehensive care for haemophiliacs trying to preserve function of the joint and improve quality of life. They have to do functional training (hydrotherapy, walking climbing stairs, cycling, etc). Osteopenia and osteoporosis can cause increased number of serious injuries and fracture after falls (Wallny, 2007). Painful haemophilic arthropathy with reduced mobility and lack of activity may lead to a reduction of bone mass. Therefore it is recommended weight-bearing physical activities or sports, but with surgery to mobilize the patient. Calcium and vitamin D supplementation are recommended (Kovacs, 2008). Secondary prophylaxis based on two to three infusions of factor concentrates per week in adult patients with haemophilia and with few older patients ≥ 65 years in small retrospective studies showed marked reduction in frequency of bleeding (Tagliaferri, 2008) but athropathy is worsening. Prophylaxis in elderly persons with haemophilia is justified and whenever possible to carry out it is improving their quality of life.

2.1.2 Chronic blood borne infections

Chronic viral infections such as HIV, hepatitis B (HBV) and hepatitis C (HCV) virus are still prevalent in a subgroup of adult haemophilia patients. It is also important to emphasis the risk of development of liver cancer on the background of chronic HCV infection; particularly with genotype 1 and HIV confection, who failed to achieve a sustained viral response with pegylated interferon and ribavirin (Posthouwer, 2007). Many of them will develop liver cirrhosis and subsequent hepatocellular carcinoma (HCC) (Posthouwer, 2007, Konkle, 2009, Siboni, 2009). Hepatocellular cancer is the most prevalent cancer in the older haemophilia patients. Therefore, surveillance program with periodic ultrasound screening is recommended to detect HCC earlier in people with haemophilia and cirrhosis. Therefore, close surveillance with gastroenterologists in collaboration with hematologist should be carried out to prevent such bleeding complications.

In HIV-infected hemophilic patients, combined antiretroviral therapy (cART) significantly improved survival rate comparing to period before the introduction of this treatment in the middle 1990s. cART has also reduced the previously frequent incidence of non-Hodgkin lymphomas (Ragni, 1993, Wilde, 2002). However, cART increases the risk of the metabolic syndrome, diabetes, renal insufficiency, and atherosclerotic cardiovascular disease in non-hemophilia patients (Lundgren et al., 2008). It is likely to suspect that cART will induce the same long-term complications among HIV-infected elderly patients with hemophilia, although there are very rare data about the long-term outcome of such patient subgroup.

Moreover, chronic viral infections such as HCV and HIV can also alter the complex inflammatory process of atherosclerosis and coronary heart disease by itself. Checking serum lipid, glucose, and creatinine at regular intervals is suggested.
In HIV-infected hemophilic patients, combined antiretroviral therapy (cART) significantly improved survival rate comparing to period before the introduction of this treatment in the middle 1990s. cART has also reduced the previously frequent incidence of non-Hodgkin lymphomas (Ragni, 1993, Wilde, 2002). However, cART increases the risk of the metabolic syndrome, diabetes, renal insufficiency, and atherosclerotic cardiovascular disease in non-hemophilia patients (Lundgren, 2008). It is likely to suspect that cART will induce the same long-term complications among HIV-infected elderly patients with haemophilia, although there are very rare data about the long-term outcome of such patient subgroup. Moreover, chronic viral infections such as HCV and HIV can also alter the complex inflammatory process of atherosclerosis and coronary heart disease by itself. Therefore, checking serum lipid, glucose, and creatinine at regular intervals is suggested.

2.1.3 Inhibitors

Data from large nationwide haemophilia population (Darby, 2004) provided estimates of the rate of development of inhibitors and showed the cumulative risk of haemophilia A inhibitors at 50 years is 30% and 36% at 75 years. Patients with milder forms of haemophilia may develop inhibitors at advanced age when they receive intensive replacement therapy preoperatively or for invasive procedures. Other risk factors for inhibitor development in mild to moderate haemophilia are certain mutations, like Arg531Cys and exposure to continuous infusion of factor concentrate (Eckhart, 2009).
The treatment of acute bleeding in older severe haemophilia A patients with inhibitors is administration of activated prothrombin concentrate (APCC) and recombinant factor VIIa. Rapid control of bleeding is the key to reducing bleeding complications and therebay preserving joint and musculoskeletal function in haemophilia patients with inhibitors (Šalek, 2011). Risk of thrombotic complication with bypassing agents is a question especially with advanced age. There are a few articles about safe administration of rFVIIa to elderly haemophilia patients with inhibitors (Rivolta, 2009; Leebeck, 2004). There is just one report about the successful immune tolerance induction (ITI) in one old haemophilia patient (60-years old) and high responding inhibitors (Rivolta, 2009). Review article published by Franchini (Franchini, 2008) found that about half of the haemophilia patients with inhibitors resistant to previous immune tolerance regimens are rescued by rituximab treatment. The highest probability to obtain complete response to rituximab was observed for adult haemophilia patients with mild to moderate haemophilia with median age of 50.5 years. Presence of inhibitors in older patient with haemophilia and their treatment represent still today a significant challenge.

2.1.4 Renal disease (urogenital disease)

Chronic kidney disease probably develops with increasing prevalence among older people with hemophilia because of multiple concomitant risk factors such as HIV infection and combined antiretroviral treatment, hematuria, structural renal damage, and use of antifibrinolytic drug. (Kulkarni, 2003).
Another important aspect of aging is erectile dysfunction resulting not only from the normal aging process, but also from co-morbidities such as painful chronic joint damage affecting sexual desire and conditions that affect erectile function, such as artheriosclerosis and

hypertension (Gianotten, 2009). The use of multiple drugs for the treatment may also compromise sexual function. Prostatic hypertrophy is also a frequent problem in elderly people with haemophilia. Genitourinary diseases and prostatic hypertrophy may facilitate the onset of hematuria as well.

2.1.5 Malignancy

The literature data showed clearly that liver cancer and lymphoma represent the most prevalent malignancy in haemophilia population. They are usually associated with HCV and HIV positivity. Hepatocellular carcinoma is very important cause of death among haemophiliacs with a reported standardized mortality ratio of 17.2 (Plug, 2006) and 13.51 (Darby, 2007). Risk factors for hepatocellular carcinoma assessed in multicentre Italian study were presence of liver cirrhosis, elevated alpha fetoprotein, current HCV infection and age over 45 (Tradati, 1998). There are many studies which do not found an increased incidence of other malignancies in haemophilia compared with general population. Moreover, two population studies found a lower incidence of cancer in severe haemophilia (Walker, 1998; Darby, 2007). *In vitro* study has shown that congenital prothrombotic disorders facilitate metastasis. Haemophiliac mice form less metastasis from experimental melanomas what could be explained with less formation of thrombin (Bruggemann, 2008). It seems that congenital bleeding disorders may have a protective effect against formation of metastasis on murine cells (Langer, 2006). Elderly patients with haemophilia will develop malignancies like normal elderly population; prostate, skin and gastrointestinal cancer (Franchini, 2009).
Treatment schemes for malignant tumours in older haemophilia patients are similar to non-haemophiliac although the inherited coagulation disorder might increase the risk of bleeding during chemo and radiotherapy. Factor replacement therapy is needed for invasive diagnostic and therapeutic procedures and prophylactic factor administration is mandatory for surgery (Mannucci, 2009; Dolan, 2010). At the moment it is not completely clear how intensive replacement therapy should be in a situation of treatment carcinoma in elderly haemophiliacs. There are no recommendations about optimal treatment of elderly haemophiliac with malignancy, except some case reports (Lambert, 2008; Toyoda, 2001). Our group publish a case of 51-year old patient with severe haemophilia A with low-titre inhibitors and multiple relapsing non-melanoma skin cancer. The management of such patients could be very intriguing and require a multidisciplinary approach (Zupančić Šalek, 2009). Age indicated screening tests for malignoma of prostate and colon are justified also in the population of elderly haemophiliacs but under the cover of prophylactic treatment with factor concentrates. Very important fact about haemophilia patients is that they are usually excluded from participating in clinical trials which are evaluating new anticancer drugs because of the potential adverse effects of haemostatic system. Definitely, treatment of older haemophilia patient with malignancy is a complex issue.

2.1.6 Pain control

Pain control is extremely important for improvement quality of life among people with haemophilia, especially due to chronic joint damage. Haemophilic arthropathy and related morbidity is still present major concern among haemophilic population. Therefore, chronic pain is prevalent in the elderly people with haemophilia, and even drug addiction is not rare. Possible adverse effects of widely used paracetamol and non-steroidal anti-inflammatory drugs (NSAIDs) may become more clinically significant with aging: gastroduodenal toxicity, paracetamol-associated liver dysfunction (particularly associated

with chronic liver disease due to excessive alcohol consumption and/or viral infections), hypertension, and renal insufficiency (Davies et al., 2006). However, paracetamol is still the first choice for pain management among haemophilia patients, and when it is not effective to control pain, cyclo-oxygenase-2 (COX-2) inhibitors are preferred to NSAIDs (Mannucci, 2009). Other possibilities are narcotics such as codeine- and morphine-containing drugs (Mannucci, 2009). Moreover, additional useful option for pain control is referral to a pain management clinic, as well as pre-emptive physiotherapy and hydrotherapy to improve joint stability.

2.1.7 Cardiovascular disease in elderly patients with hemophilia

Haemophilia is reported to be protective against development of coronary heart disease due to the hypocoagulable state of such patients (Rosendaal, 1990). However, people with haemophilia could have other common risk factors for cardiovascular diseases, such as hypertension, smoking, obesity, dyslipidaemia, and diabetes. Additionally, HIV infection and cART may *per se* increase the risk for metabolic and cardiovascular disease, as it was stated earlier. Indeed, it was reported recently an increasing number of deaths in haemophilia patients as a consequence of ischemic heart disease (Plug, 2006), together with increasing prevalence of ischemic heart disease among haemophilia patients 60 years of age and older (Kulkarni, 2005). Moreover, it is important to educate haemophilia patients about the cardiovascular risk factors, and on the benefit of living a healthy lifestyle (Mannucci, 2009).

2.2 Assessment of atherosclerotic risk factors in patients with haemophilia

2.2.1 Introduction

Myocardial and cerebral infarctions are the leading causes of death around the world (Murray, 1997). Due to its public health importance, numerous studies have examined risk factors for atherosclerosis. Due to rare reports about risk factors in haemophilia patients we present data from risk assessment in haemophiliacs.

2.2.2 Subjects and methods

During a 10-year period 410 patients with haemophilia A and B were followed in National Haemophilia Centre in University Hospital. Eight died, two of infection, three of bleeding, two of liver disease and one of malignancy. None of them died due to coronary or cerebrovascular diseases and there were no drop-outs during the follow-up. Of the surviving 402 patients, 336 (84%) had haemophilia A and 66 (16%) haemophilia B. A cohort of 117 haemophilia patients who attended regular check-ups consented to participate in our risk factors study. 104 (89%) had haemophilia A and 13 (11%) haemophilia B. Control group consists of 48 age-adjusted healthy male non-haemophiliac volunteers who did not have anamnestic or clinical signs and symptoms of coronary heart disease or other complications of atherosclerosis.

Body mass index was calculated and patients were considered to have normal weight if their BMI was below 25, overweight if the BMI was 25-29.9 and obese if the BMI was 3.0 or higher (Flegal, 1998). Blood pressure was measured and according to the WHO/ISH criteria, patents were considered having arterial hypertension if their systolic blood pressure was 140 mmHg or higher, diastolic blood pressure was 90 mmHg or higher of if they were taking antihypertensive medications(WHO/ISH, 1999). Serum concentrations of glucose,

creatinine, uric acid, fibrinogen, total cholesterol, triglycerides, HDL cholesterol and LDL cholesterol were determined using standard methods and commercially available reagents (Horvat, 2003). Homocysteine concentration and lipoprotein (a) was also determined. Framingham risk index was determined as described by Grundy and co-workers (Grundy, 1999). The ten-year risk of developing coronary heart disease in individuals without symptomatic atherosclerosis is determined taking into account their sex, age, total-cholesterol, HDL-cholesterol, systolic blood pressure, treatment of arterial hypertension and smoking. Four risk levels are recognised: low, moderate, high and very high. The expected incidence of coronary and ischaemic cerebrovascular disease morbidity and mortality for patents with haemophilia was calculated as follows. The number and age for male patents discharged from Croatian hospitals with diagnosis of myocardial infarction, coronary heart disease and cerebrovascular infarction were abstracted from official publications of the Croatian Institute for Public Health (Ljubičić, 2002). Thus calculated age adjusted morbidity and mortality rates were used to determine the expected morbidity and mortality of patients with haemophilia during the 10-year observation period.

2.2.3 Results

The tested cohort did not differ from the whole group of patients with haemophilia in respect to age and haemophilia type. More patients with haemophilia than control subjects smoked (44 vrs. 33%). This difference was even more pronounced in the group of patients with severe haemophilia (46%) but did not reach statistical significance. Patients with haemophilia had slightly lower BMI than normal controls. Again this difference was more pronounced in patients with severe disease but again, did not reach statistical significance. The incidence of abnormal BMI was similar in all analysed groups. Patients with haemophilia had similar systolic but higher diastolic blood pressure than control subjects. This difference was significant for the subgroup of patients with severe disease but not for the subgroup of patients with moderate or mild disease. The incidence of diastolic hypertension was higher in the group of patients with haemophilia than in the control group. Again, this difference was highly significant for the subgroup with severe disease but barely failed to reach significance for the subgroup of patients with moderate or mild disease. The incidence of systolic hypertension was higher in the group of patients with severe disease than in the control group (Figure 1.) The difference between all subjects with haemophilia and control subjects barely failed to reach statistical significance. These data suggest that arterial hypertension is more frequent in patients with haemophilia, especially in those with severe disease.

Patients with haemophilia did not differ from control subjects in respect to blood glucose, fibrinogen, uric acid and homocysteine concentrations, but they had lower total cholesterol, triglycerides and creatinine concentrations. The difference was even more pronounced in the subgroup of patients with severe haemophilia who also had lower LDL-cholesterol than controls. Patients with mild to moderate disease had higher HDL-cholesterol than controls. The incidence of abnormal serum glucose, fibrinogen, creatinine, uric acid and homocysteine levels was similar between groups. Controls had more frequently abnormal total cholesterol, HDL-cholesterol and triglycerides concentrations than patients with haemophilia. They had also more often abnormal total-cholesterol, LDL- cholesterol and triglycerides concentrations than patients with severe disease; an abnormal HDL-cholesterol and triglycerides concentrations than patients with mild to moderate disease.

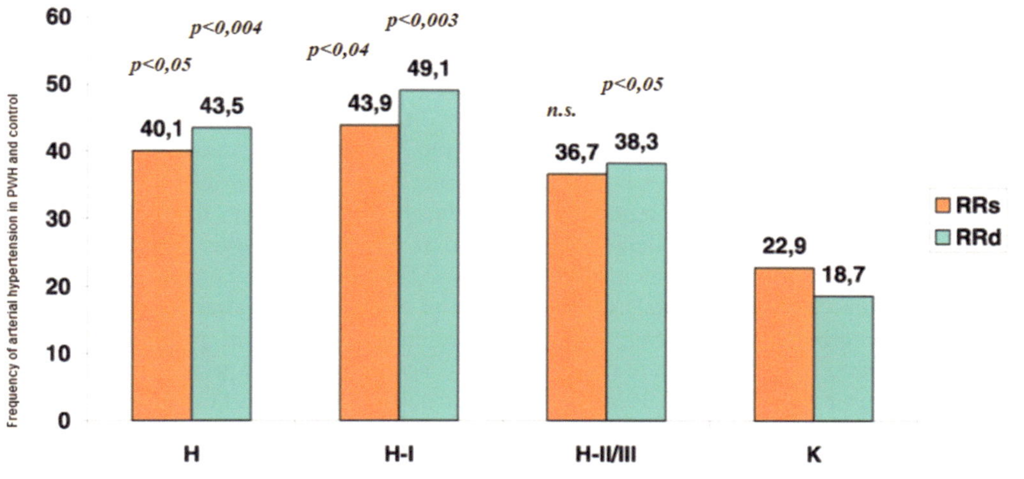

Fig. 1. Frequency of arterial hypertension in patients with haemophilia and control (Legend: red column: systolic blood pressure; blue column: diastolic blood pressure; RRs – systolic blood pressure; RRd dyastolic blood pressure, H: all haemophilia patients, H-1: severe haemophilia patients; H-II moderate haemophilia patients; H-III mild haemophilia patients)

This indicates that patients with haemophilia, especially those with severe disease have lower cholesterol and triglyceride concentrations than control subjects. In patients with mild to moderate haemophilia the increase in total cholesterol is accompanied by an increase in HDL-cholesterol, resulting in a similarly low-risk lipid profile as in those with severe disease.

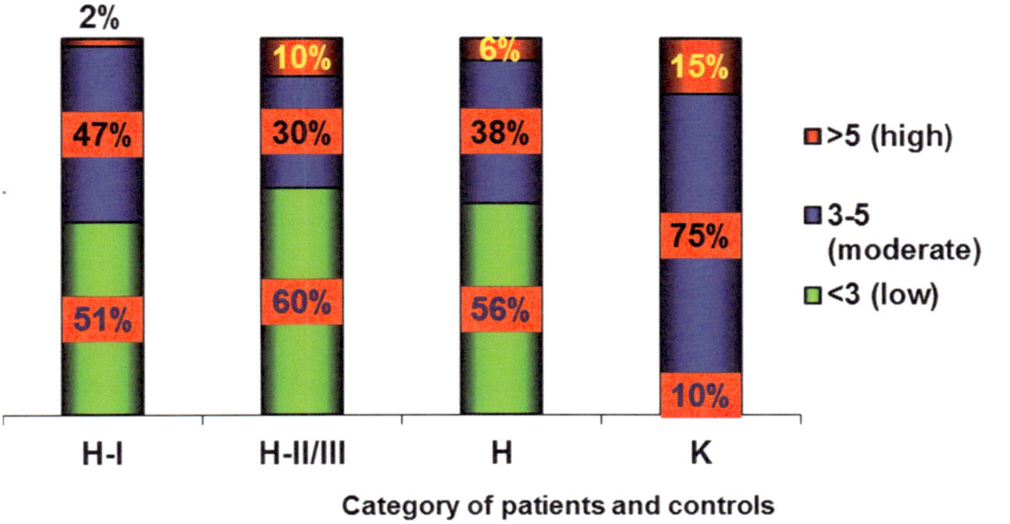

Fig. 2. Risk assessment of coronary heart disease according to LDL/HDL ratio. (Legend: H-I: severe haemophilia; H-II/III: mild and moderate haemophilia; H: all haemophilias patients and K .controls.)

Framingham risk index. The distribution of risk groups did not differ between patients with haemophilia and control subjects. However, some of the patients with severe disease had a high or very high risk of developing coronary heart disease. None such cases could be seen in the control group (Figure 2).

If the morbidity of myocardial infarction and ischaemic cerebrovascular infarction, calculated as described in "Methods" section, would be the same in patients with haemophilia as it is in the general Croatian population, during the ten-year observation period 18 patients would be expected to develop myocardial infarction and 10 ischaemic cerebrovascular infarction. However, none occurred. These differences are highly statistically significant. If the mortality of coronary heart disease, myocardial infarction or cerebrovascular infarction, calculated as described in section "Methods" , would be the same in patients with haemophilia as it is in the general Croatian population, during the ten-year observation period 8 patients would be expected to die of coronary heart disease, 4 of myocardial infarction and 4 of cerebrovascular infarction. None of them died. These differences are statistically significant. These data indicate that patients with haemophilia have a significant lower incidence of complications of atherosclerosis than the general population.

The concentration of lipoprotein (a) as well as the proportion of subjects with abnormal levels is higher in the group of patients with haemophilia than in the controls. The difference is more pronounced in the subgroup of patients with mild to moderate disease, while the difference between patients with severe haemophilia and controls fails to reach statistical significance (Figure 3).

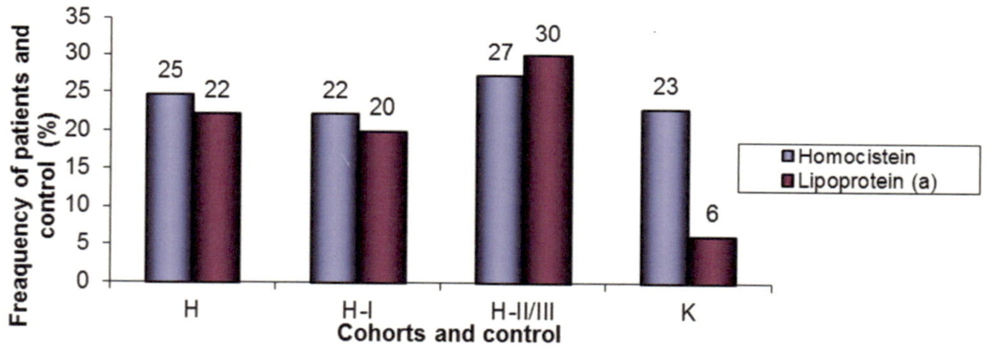

Fig. 3. Frequency of abnormal values for homocysteine and lipoprotein (a) (Legend: H-I: severe haemophilia; H-II/III: mild and moderate haemophilia; H: all haemophilia patients and K: controls.)

2.2.3.1 Risk factors

Our results suggest that patients with haemophilia smoke somewhat more frequently than the subjects from the control group or the general Croatian population. Two studies, one Dutch and the other Italian study with patients with haemophilia have reached the same conclusion (Rosendaal et al 1990; Bilora, 1999). This is most probably due to psychological changes induced by the presence of a chronic disease and the enforced sedentary life style. Our patients have s slightly lower BMI than healthy subjects. The same was found in the Dutch study. Again, this is more probably a result of reduced muscle mass in patients with haemophilia, caused by their sedentary life style, than their superior health consciousness.

The incidence of hypertension in the group of patients with haemophilia was 48%, while it was 20% in the control group. The latter incidence is surprisingly low, probably due to the fact that the control subjects had to be free from any signs and symptoms of disease due to atherosclerosis. An epidemiological study performed in 2 898 Croatian subjects found a 32% incidence of hypertension, still lower than in patients with haemophilia (Turek, 2001). The increase in blood pressure we observed was even more pronounced in patients with severe haemophilia and was already present in the youngest group aged between 18 and 29 years. This might suggest that haemophilia somehow causes hypertension. The underlying mechanisms are completely unclear and further research is needed. Renal damage is certainly not the cause.

Patients with haemophilia have more favourable lipid profiles than control subjects. Again, similar findings were obtained by Rosendaal. Lowest cholesterol levels are seen in patients with severe haemophilia. In patients with milder disease total cholesterol is increased, but so it HDL-cholesterol, resulting in a lipid profile that is still favourable than in control subjects. Since we have no reason to believe that patients with haemophilia adhere to a more healthy diet than average person, we agree with the explanation of Rosendaal and col. That this difference is due to a reduced liver synthetic capacity caused by an increased exposure to foreign proteins and transfusion related viral diseases.

Increased homocyteine levels were seen in 25 % of patients with haemophilia and 23% control subjects. These proportions are not statistically different, but are higher than those published for other populations. The reason for this is not clear.

Patient with haemophilia has increased lipoprotein (a) levels. There are reports indicating that lipoprotein (a) levels are reduced in haemophilia patients with AIDS. and that the incidence of increased lipoprotein (a) levels in children with haemophilia is not different from that observed in the general population (Matsuda et al 1994). There are no reports on the concentration of lipoprotein (a) in adult, HIV negative, patients with haemophilia. Since these concentrations are genetically determined and not influenced by diet, studies in other populations are needed to determine whether the increase is characteristic for haemophilia or specific for tested population (Scanu, 1992).

2.2.3.2 Global risk assessment

The Framingham risk index is a reliable predictor of the ten-year risk for the development of coronary heart disease for persons who did not have prior complications of atherosclerosis (Grundy, 1998). it is used in USA guidelines for arterial hypertension and hypercholesterolemia treatment. It is still one of the best and most validated global risk assessment tools for risk factors for coronary heart disease in patients with haemophilia. According to the Framingham risk index, patients with haemophilia are similar to the control group. While the global assessment is similar, there are important differences in risk profiles. Patients with haemophilia have more favourable lipid profiles, but tend to smoke and have arterial hypertension more frequent than control subjects. Still, some of the patients with severe haemophilia have high risk features, while none such subjects were found in the control group. If the difference in newly recognized risk factors, such as lipoprotein (a) levels, would be taken into account, the increase in risk in the haemophilia group would be even more pronounced.

2.2.3.3 Coronary heart disease and cerebrovascular morbidity and mortality

The expected coronary and cerebrovascular morbidity and mortality in the group of patients with haemophilia is probably underestimated. The difference between the expected and

observed coronary heart disease and cerebrovascular morbidity and mortality in patients with haemophilia is highly significant. The same phenomenon was observed by other authors in other countries. This indicates that patients with haemophilia have a reduced risk of developing and dying of myocardial infarction, coronary heart disease and ischaemic cerebrovascular infarction.

2.2.4 Haemophilia and atherosclerosis

The reduction of complications of atherosclerosis in patients with haemophilia is not due to a reduction in known risk factors. It is tempting to assume that the inability to produce a stable thrombus, i.e. haemophilia itself, is the cause. Our results and the published data suggest that haemophilia protects patients against atherosclerosis and complications but it is still not clear whether this is due only to the lack of thromboembolic incidents occurring late in the process of atherogenesis.

2.3 Osteoporosis

2.3.1 Introduction

Since the world's population is ageing, osteoporosis has become one of the major socioeconomic problems in the western world. As a consequence of reduced bone mass and decline in neuromuscular function, the risk of osteoporotic fractures is rising with the advancing age, both in men and in women. Fractures of the spine, proximal femur and a distal forearm are described as typical for osteoporosis; nevertheless, almost all types of bone fractures are increased in patients with reduced bone mineral mass. Many factors influence bone mass accumulation in early life, and maintenance of that mass in adult age. including genetic factors, hormonal status, physical activity and calcium intake. Besides genetics, which has the highest impact on bone mass accumulation and maintenance, the changes of hormonal status in ageing woman have been described to have strong impact on bone mineral mass.

2.3.2 Osteoporosis in haemophilia patients

Recently, bone mineral mass has become an issue of interest in patients with haemophilia. Although there are only sparse data about osteoporotic fractures in haemophilia patients, we can expect increase in number of osteoporotic fractures in the future due to ageing of haemophilia population. Morbidity and mortality of osteoporotic fractures in haemophilia patients are very high, and those patients need special care (Rodriguez-Merchan, 2002.). Moreover, it has been shown that patients with haemophilia and reduced bone mass have lower quality of life (Khawaji, 2010.). Studies addressing bone mineral mass in haemophilia patients mainly focused on patients with severe haemophilia. Because haemophilia is rare disease, total number of studied patients is relatively low.

2.3.3 Incidence of reduced bone mass in haemophilia patients

The incidence of reduced mineral bone mass among patients with haemophilia differs between studies. Our results, in a study where we evaluated 58 patients with haemophilia, showed reduced bone mass in 56% of patients with haemophilia. Those results are comparable with findings of Nair, who described reduced bone mass in 50% of patients with severe haemophilia (Nair, 2007). On the other hand, some authors showed reduced bone mass in 86% patients with severe and moderate haemophilia (FVIII<3%) (Katsarou,

2009), and in 70% of patients with severe haemophilia (Gerstner, 2009, Wallny, 2007). The reason for difference between those results is uncertain.

The data about incidence of reduced bone mineral mass in patients with moderate or mild haemophilia are sparse. Our results showed increased loss of bone mineral density in patients with mild and moderate haemophilia (FVIII>1%). In comparison of bone mass between patients with severe and patients with mild or moderate haemophilia, the difference was noted in values of bone mineral density measured at femoral neck, representing cortical bone, where patients with mild and moderate haemophilia had higher values (Boban, unpublished data). See Figure 4.

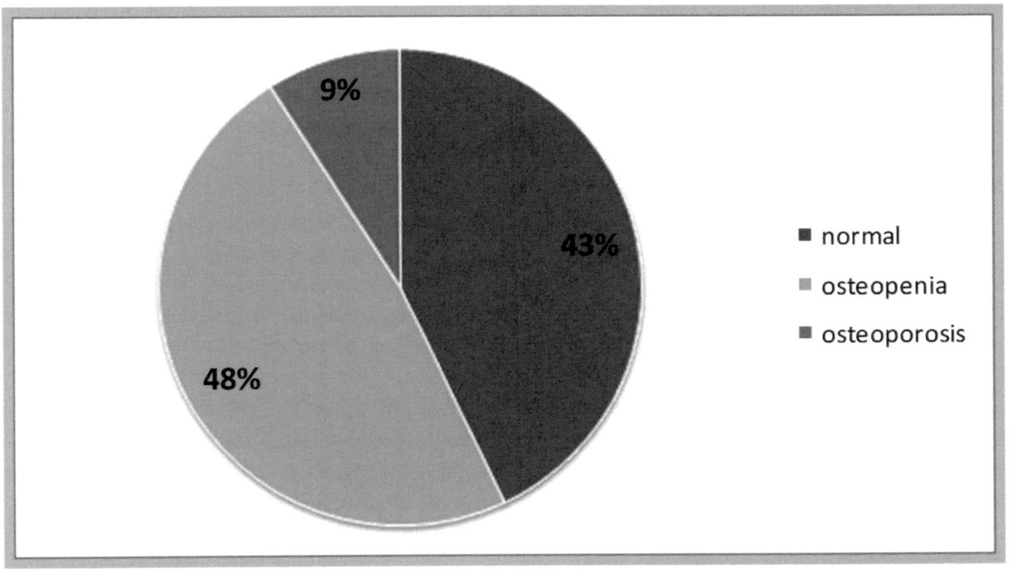

Fig. 4. Prevalence of osteopenia and osteoporosis in patients with haemophilia.

2.3.4 Physical activity

Several risk factors for developing osteoporosis in patients with haemophilia have been recognized. Besides genetics, reduction of physical activity during childhood and adult age has been suggested to have major impact on bone metabolism in haemophilia patients. However, the exact pathogenesis of developing reduced bone mineral mass in haemophilia patients is still obscure. Patients with haemophilia seem to achieve lower peak bone mineral mass when compared to healthy controls. In favour of this hypothesis, studies showed reduced bone mineral density among children with severe haemophilia (Barnes, 2004, Abdelrazik , 2007., Nair, 2007., Tlacuilo-Parra, 2008.). The major impact on bone formation during childhood and adolescents has physical activity and, moreover, weight-bearing exercises. Patients with haemophilia avoid physical activity due to acute bleedings into joints, chronic pain, development of arthropathy, and fear of possible injury. The study showed that 77% of young haemophiliacs are inactive; with the high correlation of inactivity and reduced bone mass (Tlacuilo-Parra, 2008).

The role of physical activity in maintaining or even improving bone mass in adult age is questionable. The only study that evaluated influence of physical activity on bone mass in

adult haemophilia patient did not show any correlation between those two parameters (Khawaji, 2010.). However, we must point out that patients enrolled in the mentioned study had normal bone mineral mass.

2.3.5 Joint status and prophylactic therapy

The strong relationship has been established between reduced bone mass and joint status in young patients with haemophilia (Abdelrazik, 2007), as well as among adult haemophiliacs (Nair, 2007., Katsarou, 2009.). Joint status was evaluated using clinical score as described by the Orthtopedic Advisory Council of the World Federation of Haemophilia (Rodriguez-Merchan EC, 2003.) and by the Pettersson scores (Pettersson, 1994). Total joint score had independent prognostic value for development of bone loss (Nair, 2007., Katsarou, 2009). In our study number of target joints was evaluated as a prognostic factor for development of bone loss. No correlation was found between bone mass and number of target joints (Boban, unpublished data).

Prophylactic therapy, however, seems to prevent bone mineral loss. Prophylactic therapy significantly reduces the risk of developing haemophilic arthropathy, thus avoiding immobilization, crippling, and chronic pain (Manco-Johnson, 2007). Young patients with haemophilia that received prophylactic therapy had only slightly reduced bone mass (Barnes, 2004). Moreover, adult patients with haemophilia that received prophylactic treatment since childhood had bone mass comparable to patients with mild haemophilia (Khawaji, 2009.).

2.3.6 Inhibitors

Patients with inhibitors have significantly more joint pain with clinically and radiological worse orthopaedic status than patient without inhibitors (Morfini, 2007). Therefore, due to pathogenesis of osteoporosis in patient with haemophilia, they were expected to have lower bone mass than patients without inhibitors. Data about bone mineral mass in haemophilia patients with inhibitors in the literature are sparse. Only very few patients with inhibitors were evaluated. The study on 6 patients showed that patients with increased bone loss were statistically more likely to have a history of factor inhibitor (Gerstner, 2009). We have evaluated 9 patients with severe haemophilia and inhibitors. The results showed no difference in bone mineral mass between patients with severe haemophilia and with and without inhibitors. The discrepancy between those two studies may be explained by different treatment approaches. Moreover, in our study, no difference was found in number of target joints between patients with and without inhibitors, which can suggest effective treatment (Boban, unpublished data).

2.3.7 Infection with hepatitis C

Infection with hepatitis C virus (HCV) has been recognized as a risk factor for development of increased bone loss. HCV infection can lead to chronic liver disease, and consequently to increased bilirubin levels, hypogonadims and abnormalities in vitamin D metabolism, which can have negative influence on bone turnover (Olsson, 1994, Schiefke, 2005). Influence of HCV infection on bone loss in patients with haemophilia is still unclear. Two studies (Nair, 2007, Barnes, 2004) found no significant difference in bone mass between HCV positive and negative patients. On the other hand, Wallny showed significantly lower bone mass in heamophilia patients that were HCV positive (Wallny, 2007). According to our

study, HCV infection had no influence on bone mineral mass in patients with haemophilia. Nevertheless, slight difference was seen in group of patients with mild and moderate haemophilia, where we discovered negative influence of HCV infection on bone mineral (Boban, unpublished data).

2.3.8 Quantitative ultrasound of the heel

Dual energy X-ray absorptionmetry (DXA) is the golden standard for measurement of bone mineral mass. Quantitative ultrasound (QUS) of the heel is emerging as a new, low cost screening technique that is able to identify risk of osteoporotic fractures. The QUS parameters, BUA (broadband sound attenuation) and SOS (speed of sound) depend not only on mineral bone mass, but also on micro architecture and physical properties of bone tissue. A number of studies showed that the values of parameters measured with QUS are lower in woman with the history of osteoporotic fractures, regardless of the bone mineral density determined by DXA (Hernandez, 2004, Gluer, 2004). Thus, QUS parameters are independent risk indicator for hip fractures. Our study observed reduced bone properties among patients with severe hemophilia determined by QUS. On the other hand, patients with mild and moderate hemophilia had QUS values comparable to healthy controls. Sensitivity and specificity of QUS in finding reduced bone mineral density was 70,4% and 64%, respectively. However, among studied population we observed no history of osteoporotic fractures. Therefore, we could not assess QUS as the method for identifying risk of osteoporotic fractures in patients with haemophilia (Boban, unpublished data).

2.3.9 Haemophilia and bone mineral density

Assessment of frequency of osteoporosis/osteopenia in patients with haemophilia A/B has been undertaken in National Haemophilia Centre. Results showed that patients with haemophilia have high risk of developing osteoporosis and osteopenia, which is dependent on severity of haemophilia, but not on presence of FVIII inhibitors or hepatitis C infection. Quantitative ultrasound of the heel, after modification of T- cut off values, showed high sensitivity and specificity for detection of reduced bone mineral density in haemophilia patients.

3. Conclusion

The improved diagnosis and comprehensive care of patients with hemophilia around the world have introduced the new problems of an aging patients with hemophilia and other co-morbidities. It is obvious that population of people with hemophilia is getting older, approaching life expectancy that of the general male population; at least in countries that can afford regular replacement therapy with coagulation factor concentrates.

Such improvement of life expectancy among people with hemophilia is due to several factors: advances in hemophilia replacement treatment, comprehensive care, home treatment and prophylaxis, as well as due to advances in general health care improvement.

Two investigations have been set in Hemophilia Centre. The first one was conducted about the frequency of classical risk factors of coronary heart disease in patients with haemophilia A and B as well as new risk actors - homocysteine and lipoprotein (a).

The frequencies of atherosclerotic complications are less expressed in haemophilia patients than expected from the data of the normal Croatian population

The results of investigated risk factors of CHD in patients' with haemophilia reveal the importance to follow up in spite of the protection of haemophilia in clinical manifestations of atherosclerosis.

Recently, Biere-Rafi (Biere-Rafi, 2011) also published data about cardiovascular risk assessment in haemophilia patients. They found that the number of hemophiliacs with hyperglycaemie (24%) and hypertension (51%) was higher than in the controls. It is comparable with our results that hemophiliacs have more arterial hypertension than the control group. Also, they have lower level of low-density lipoprotein (LDL) than control what is also comparable with our results.

Considering high prevalence of patients with cardiovascular risk factors, active screening for these factors is recommended.

The second investigation assessed the frequency of osteoporosis/osteopenia in patients with haemophilia A/B (see 2.3.9.).

The aging haemophilia population will have much co-morbidities like older general population, however with specific complex requirements due to bleeding tendency. There are well established guidelines of care for the younger people with hemophilia, but it is necessary to have guidelines of care for aging hemophilia patients as well.

4. References

Abdelrazik, N.; El-Ziny, M.; Rabea, H. (2007). Evaluation of bone mineral density in children with hemophilia: Mansoura University children hospital (MUCH) experience, Mansoura, Egypt. *Hematology, Oct;12(5): 431-7.*

Barnes, C WP.; Egan, B.; Speller, T.; Cameron, F.; Jones, G.; Ekert, H.; Monagle, P. (2004.) Reduced bone density among children with severe hemophilia. *Pediatrics, Aug;114 (2): e177-81.*

Biere-Rafi, S.; Baarslag, MA.; Peters, M.; Kruip, MJHA.; Kraaijenhagen, RA.; Heijer, MD.; Buller, HR. and Kamphuisen, PW. (2011) Cardiovascular risk assessment in haemophilia patients. *Thrombosis and Haemostasis. 105:274-278.*

Bilora,F.; dei Rossi,C.; Girolami,B.; Casonato, A.; Zanon,E.; Bertomoro, A.; Girolami, A.(1999). Do haemophilia A and von Willebrand disease protect against carotid atherosclerosis? A comparative study between coagulopathies and normal subjects by means of carotid echo-colour Doppler scan. *Clin Appl Thormb Haemost 5:232-235*

Birch C, La F. (2008) Haemophilia, clinical and genetic aspects. Urbana: University of Illinois, 1937.

Bruggemann, LW.; Versteeg, HH.; Nieres, TM.; Reitsma, PH.; and Spek, CA. (2008) Experimental melanoma metastasis in lungs of mice with congenital coagulation disorders. *J Cell mol Med 12(6B): 2622-2627.*

Chorba, TL.; Holman, RC.; Clarke, MJ.; Evatt, BL. (2001) Effects of HIV infection on age and cause of death for persons with Haemophilia A in the United States. *Am J Hematol. 66:229-240.*

Dalldorf,FD.; Taylor,RE.; Blatt,PM. (1981) Artheriosclerosis in severe haemophilia. *Arch Pathol Lab Med. 10:652-654.*

Darby, SC.; Keeling, DM.; Spooner, RJ. et al. (2004) UK Haemophilia Centre Doctors' Organization. The incidence of factor VIII and factor IX inhibitors in the hemophilia population of the UK and their effect on subsequent mortality, 1977-99. *J Thromb Haemost.*2:*1047-1054.*

Darby, SC.; Kan, SW.; Spooner, RJ.; Giangrande, PLF.; Hill, FGH.; Hay, CRM.; Lee, CA.; Ludlam, CA.; and Williams, M. (2007) Mortality rates, life expectancy, and causes of death in people with hemophilia A or B in the United Kingdom who were not infected with HIV. *Blood, 110:815-825.*

Davies, NM.; Reynolds, JK.; Undeberg, MR.; Gates, BJ.; Ohgami, Y.; Vega-Villa, KR. (2006) Minimizing risks of NSAIDs: cardiovascular, gastrointestinal and renal. *Expert Rev Neurother. 6(11):1643- 1655.*

Dolan, G. (2010) The challenge of an ageing hemophilia population. *Haemophilia. 16 (Suppl.5), 11-16.*

Eckhart, Cl.; Menke, LA.; van Ommen, CH., et al. (2009).Intensive peri-operative use of factor VIII and the Arg593cys mutation are risk factors for inhibitor development. *J Thromb Haemost.7:9228-929.*

Flegal, KM.; Carroll, MD.; Kuczmarski, RJ.; Johnson, CL. (1998). Overweight and obesity in the United States. Prevalence and trends, 1960-1994. *Int J Obes. 22:39-47.*

Franchini, M.; Mengoli, C.; Lippi, G.; Targher, G.; Montagnana, M.; Salvagno, GL.; Zaffanello, M.; & Cruciani, M.(2008) Immune tolerance with rituximab in congenital haemophilia with inhibitors: a systematic literature review based on individual patients' analysis. *Haemophilia 14, 903-912.*

Franchini, M;, Manzato, F.; Salvagno, G.L.; et al. (2009). Prophylaxis in congenital hemophilia with inhibitors: the role of recombinant activated factor VII. *Semin Thromb Hemost, 35:814-819.*

Franchini, M.; Lippi, G.; Montagnana, M.; Targher, G.; Zaffanello, M.; Salvagno, GL.; Rivolata, GF.; Perna, C.D.; and Tagliaferri, A. (2009) Haemophilia and cancer: a new challenge for hemophilia centers . *Cancer Treatment Reviews, 35, 374-377.*

Franchini, M.; and Mannuccio ,PM. (2009) Co-morbidities and quality of life in elderly persons with haemophilia. *British J Haematology, 148;522-533.*

Franchini,M.; Tagliaferri, A.; Mannucci, PM. (2007) The management of haemophilia in elderly patients. *Clin Interv Aging 2:361-368.*

Gerstner, G. D. M.; Tom A, Worman ,C.; Schultz, W.; Recht, M.; Stopeck, AT. (2009).Prevalence and risk factors associated with decreased bone mineral density in patients with haemophilia. *Haemophilia. Mar;15(2): 559-65.*

Gianotten, WL.; Heijnen, L. (2009) Haemophilia, aging and sexuality. *Haemophilia.* 15(1):55-62.

Gringeri,A.; Mantovani, L.; & von Mackensen, S. (2006) Quality of life assessment in clinical in haemophilia treatment. *Haemophilia. 12 (Suppl.3), 22-29.*

Grundy, SM., Balady,GJ.; Criqui,MH.; et al. (1998). Primary prevention of coronary heart disease:guidance from Framingham. *Circulation 97:1876-1887*

Grundy, SM. (1999). Primary prevention of coronary heart disease: Integrating risk assessment with intervention. *Circulation 100:988-98.*

Guidelines Subcommittee (1999). World Health Organisation - International Society of Hypertension guidelines for the management of hypertension. *J Hypertens 7:151-83.*

Gluer, CC.; Eastell, R.; Reid, DM.; et al. (2004). Association of five quantitative ultrasound devices and bone densitometry with osteoporotic vertebral fractures in population-based sample: The OPUS study. *J Bone Miner Res 19:782-793.*

Hernandez, JL. ; Marin, F. ; Gonzalez-Macias, J. ; et al. (2004). Discriminative capacity of calcaneal quantitative ultrasound and fracture risk factors in postmenopausal women with osteoporotic fractures. *Calcif Tissue. Int 74:357-365.*

Hoffman, C.; Rice, D.; and Sung, HY. (1995) Persons with chronic conditions, their - and costs. *JAMA 276;1473-1479.*

Horvat, D.; Zrinski-Topić, R.; Bilić, A.; Stavljenić-Rukavina, A. (2003). Determination of HDL-C concentration: the importance of hypertrigliceridaemia for the choice of the method. *Biochemia Medica, 3-4:137-43 (In Croatian)*

Katsarou, O T E.; Chatzismalis Provelengios, S.; Adraktas, T.; Hadjidakis, D.; Kouramba, A.; Karafoulidou,A. (2009.) Increased bone resorption is implicated in the pathogenesis of bone loss in hemophiliacs: correlations with hemophilic arthropathy and HIV. *Annals of Hematology,* Jun 2.

Konkle, BA.; Kessler, C.; Aledort L, et al. Emerging clinical concerns in the ageing haemophilia patient. *Haemophilia.* 2009;15(6):1197-1209.

Khawaji, M A K.; Berntorp, E. (2009). Long-term prophylaxis in severe haemophilia seems to preserve bone mineral density. *Haemophilia, Jan;15(1): 261-6.*

Khawaji, M.A.J.; Akesson, K.; Berntorp, E. (2010). Physical activity for prevention of osteoporosis in patients with severe haemophilia on long-term prophylaxis. *Haemophilia,* 1-7.

Khawaji, M.; Astermark, J.; Von Mackensen, S.; et al. (2011). Bone density and health-related quality of life in adult patients with severe haemophilia. *Haemophilia, Mar;17(2):304-11.*

Kovacs, CS. (2008) Hemophilia, low bone mass, and osteopenia/osteoporosis. *Transf Apher Sci. 38:1079-1083.*

Kulkarni, R.; Soucie, JM.; and Evatt, B. (2003). Hemophilia Surveillance System Project Investigators. Renal disease among males with haemophilia. *Haemophilia. 9;703-710.*

Kulkarni, R.; Soucie, JM.; Evatt, B.(2003). Renal disease among males with haemophilia. *Haemophilia 9(6):703-710.*

Kulkarni, R.; Soucie, JM.; Evatt, BL; (2005). Hemophilia Surveillance System Project Investigators. Prevalence and risk factors for heart disease among males with hemophilia. *Am J Hematol. 79(1):36-42.*

Lambert, C.; Deneys,V. ; Pothen, D.&Hermans, C. (2008) Safety of bevacizumab in mild haemophilia B. *Thrombosis and Haemostasis, 99. 963-964.*

Langer, F.; Amirkhosravi, A.; Ingersoll, SB. et al. (2006) Experimental metastasis and primary tumor growth in mice with haemophilia A. *J Thromb Haemost. 4(5): 1056-1062.*

Leebeck, FWG.; Kappers-Klunne, MC.; & Jie, KSG. (2004) Effective and safe use of recombinant factor VIIa (Novo Seven) in elderly mild haemophilia A patients with high-titre antibodies against factor VIII. *Haemophilia, 10, 250-253.*

Lundgren, JD.; Battegay, M.; Behrens, G; et al. (2008).European AIDS Clinical Society (EACS) guidelines on the prevention and management of metabolic diseases in HIV. *HIV Med. (2):72-81.*

Ljubičić, M.; Kuzman,M. et al (2002) Croatian health-statistic annals for year 2002. Croatian Institute for Public Health, Zagreb, 2002

Mannucci, PM.; Schutgens, REG.; Santagostino, E. and Mauser-Bunschoten, EP. (2009) How I treat age-related morbidities in elderly persons with hemophilia. *Blood. 114:5256-5263.* Manco-Johnson, MJ.; Abshire, TC.; Shapiro, et al. (2007) Prophylaxis versus

episodic treatment to prevent joint disease in boys with severe haemophilia. *N Engl J Med. 357;535-544.*

Matsuda, J.; Saitoh,N., Gohecki, K.; Gotoh,M.; Tsukamoto, M. (1994) Low serum lipoprotein (a) and beta-2-lipoprotein I levels in HIV−1 positive haemophiliacs. *Ann Hematol. 68:315-316.*

Mejia-Carvajal, C.; Czapek, EE.; and Valentino, LA. (2006) Life expectancy in hemophilia outcome. *Journal of Thrombosis and Haemostasis. 4, 507-509.*

Morfini, M., Haya, S., Tagariello, G., et al. (2007). European Study on Orthopaedic Status of haemophilia patientns with inhibitors. *Haemophilia.* 13, *606-612.*

Murray, CJ.; & Lopez, AD. (1997) Global mortality, disability, and the contribution of risk factors: global burden of disease study. *Lancet. 349:1436-1442.*

Nair, APJF.; Ghosh, K.; Madkaikar, M.; Shrikhande, M.; Nema.; M. (2007). Osteoporosis in young haemophiliacs from western India. *American Journal of* Hematolology. *Jun;82(6): 453-7.*

Nilsson, IM.; Berntorp, E.; Lofqvist, T. and Pettrsson, H. (1992) Twenty-five years , experience of prophylactic in severe haemophilia A and B. *J Intern Med. 232-:25-32.* Oldenburg, J.; Dolan, G.; Lemm, G. (2009) Haemophilia care then, now and in the future. *Haemophilia. 15 (Suppl 1) :1-2.*

Olsson, R., Johansson, C., Lindstedt, G., et al. (1994) Risk factors for bone loss in chronic active hepatitis and primary biliary cirrhosis. *Scandinavian Journal of Gastroenterology, 29:753-756.*

Pettersson H (1994). Can joint damage be quantified? *Semin Hematol. 31 (Suppl 2):1-4.*

Philipp ,C. (2010). The aging patient with haemophilia: complications, comorbidities and management issues. *Hematology 191-196.*

Plug, I.; Van Der Bom,JG.; & Peters,M.; et al. (2006) Mortality and causes of death in patients with haemophilia, 1992-2001: a prospective cohort study. *J Thromb Haemost. 4;510-516.*

Posthouwer, D.; Makris, M.; Yee, TT.; et al. (2007). Progression to end-stage liver disease in patients with inherited bleeding disorders and hepatitis C: an international, multicenter cohort study. *Blood. 09(9):3667-3671.*

Posthouwer D, Yee TT, Makris M, et al. (2007)Antiviral therapy for chronic hepatitis C in patients with inherited bleeding disorders: an international, multicenter cohort study. *J Thromb Haemost. 5(8):1624-1629.*

Ragni, MV.; Belle, SH.; Jaffe, RA.; et al. (1993) Acquired immunodeficiency syndrome-associated non- Hodgkin's lymphomas and other malignancies in patients with hemophilia. *Blood.81(7): 1889-1897.*

Rivolta, GF.; Di Perna, C.; Franchini, M.; Riccardi, F.; Ippolito, L.; Lombardi, M. & Tagliaferi, A. (2010) Successful Immune tolerance induction with factor VIII/von Willebrand factor concentrate in an elderly patient with severe haemophilia A and a high responder inhibitor. *Blood Trans. 8;66-68.*

Rivolta, GF.; Di Perna, C.; Franchini, M.; Ippolito, L. ; Maurizio, S.; Rocci, A. & Tagliaferri, A. (2009) Management of coronary artery disease in a severe haemophilia patient with high titre inhibitor and anaphylaxis. *Haemophilia 15, 1159-1179.*

Rodriguez-Merchan, EC. (2010). Bone fractures in the haemophilic patient. *Haemophilia,* 8, 104–111.

Rosendaal, FR.; Briët, E.; Stibbe, J.; van Herpen, G.; Leuven, JA.; Hofman,A.; Vandenbroucke, JP. (1990). Haemophilia protects against ischaemic heart disease: a study of risk factors. *Br J Haematol. 75(4):525-30.*

Salek, ZS, Elezovic, I. et al. (2011).The need for speed in the managenet of haemophilia patients with inhibitors. *Haemophilia,* 17: 95-102.

Salomon, O.; Steinberg, DM.; Darlik, R., Rosenberg,N; Zivelin,A.;Tamarin, I.; Ravid , B. & Seligsoh, U.(2002) Inherited factor XI deficiency confers no protection against myocardial infarction. *Thromb Haemost. 1:658-661.*

Scalone, L.; Mantovani, LG.; Mannucci, PM.; Gringeri, A. and COCIS Study Investigators. (2006) Quality of life is associated to the orthopaedic status in hemophiliac patients with inhibitors. *Haemophilia. 12, 154-162.*

Scanu, AM.(1992) Lipoprotein (a). A gentic risk factor for premature coronary heart disease. *J am Med Assoc. 267;3326-3329.*

Schiefke, I., Fach, A., Wiedmann, M., et al. (2005). Reduced bone mineral density and altered bone turnover markers in patients with non-cirrhotic hepatitis B or C infection. *World Journal of Gastroenterology, 11:1843-1847.*

Siboni, SM.; Mannucci, PM.; Gringeri, A. et al. (2009) Health status and quality of life of elderly persons with severe -hemophilia born before the advent of modern replacement therapy. *J Thromb Haemost. 7:780-786.*

Tagliaferri, A. (2009) Hemophilia and Cancer: A New challenge for hemophilia centers. *Cancer Treatment Reviews. 35:374-377.*Tradati, F.; Colombo, M.; Mannucci, PM. et al. (1998) A Prospective multicenter study of hepatocellular carcinoma in Italian haemophiliacs with chronic hepatitis C. *Blood, 91 (4):1173-1177.*

Tagliaferri, A.; Rivolta, GF.; Ioro,A. et al. (2010) Mortality and causes of death in Italian persons with haemophilia. *Haemophilia. 16:437-466.*

Tlacuilo-Parra A, M.-Z. R., Tostado-Rabago, N., Esparza-Flores MA, Lopez-Guido B, Orozco-Alcala J. (2008). Inactivity is a risk factor for low bone mineral density among haemophilic children. *British Journal of Haematology,* Mar;140(5): 562-7.

Toyoda, H.; Fukuda,Y.; Yokozaki, S.; Hayashi, K.; Saito, H. & Takamatsu, J. (2001) Safety and complications of interventional radiology for hepatocellular carcinoma in patients with haemophilia and cirrhosis. *British Journal of Haematology. 112, 1071-1073.*

Turek, S.; Rudan,I.; Smolej-Narančić, N et al.(2001) A large cross-sectional study of health attitudes, knowledge, behavior and risks in the post-war Croatian population (The first Croatian health project) *Coll Anthropol 25:77-96.*

Walker, IR.; and Julian, JA. (1998) Association of Hemophilia Clinic Directors of Canada. Causes of death in Canadians with haemophilia 1980 -1995. *Haemophilia 4 (5):714-720.*

Wallny, TA. S. D.; Oldenburg, J.; Nicolay, C.; Ezziddin, S.; Pennekamp, PH.; Stoffel-Wagner, B.; Kraft, CN. (2007). Osteoporosis in haemophilia - an underestimated comorbidity? *Haemophilia, Jan;13(1): 79-84.*

Wilde JT, Lee CA, Darby SC, et al. (2002). The incidence of lymphoma in the UK haemophilia population between 1978 and 1999. *AIDS. 16(13): 1803-1807.*

Zupancic Salek, S.; Radman, I.; Pulanic, D.; Pasic, A.; Nola, M.; and Labar. B. (2009) Treatment of multiple relapsing non-melanoma skin cancer in a patient with severe hemophilia A. *Tumori,95:115-118.*